EAT BY COLOR

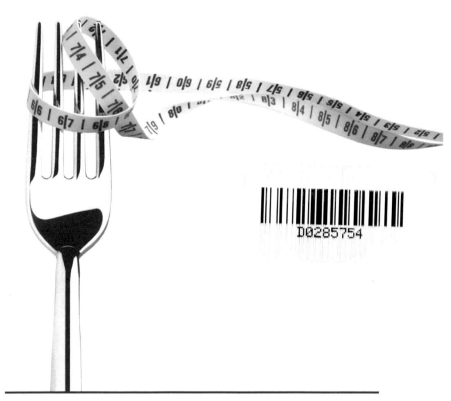

If you can paint by number, you can **EAT BY COLOR** and

lose weight

Raymond M. Binkowski

FORWARD

The amount of information on nutrition, health, and exercise is very daunting. There are endless sources of information available. Today so much information is available that finding answers results is information overload.

Complicating matters are the number of fad diets and exercise equipment hitting the market daily. There seems to be a new "get results yesterday" diet or infomercial everyday. Through the misinformation and confusion there are products and diets that work. Some "good" information can be found in every diet. The key is finding that "good" and making it work for you.

The goal of this book is to cut through the clever marketing and shine a spotlight on the information you need to be successful in your health, fitness and weight loss goals. Most importantly, this approach makes losing fat and being healthy as simple as possible. As simple as children's paint by number!

Thanks to Dr. Rod Caughron and Karen Wickersham for editing this book. Thanks to Nancy and everyone at Le Print Express for all the design and formatting. Cover art by MorningStar Media Group Ltd.

Dedicated to my wife, daughter, and mom.

For more information about Eat by Color, go to facebook.com/EatbyColor.

In memory of

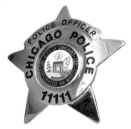

DISCLAIMER

Raymond M. Binkowski is not a physician or registered dietitian. The contents of this book should not be taken as medical advice. It is not intended to diagnose, treat, cure, or prevent any health problem – nor is it intended to replace the advice of a physician. Always consult your physician or qualified health professional on any matters regarding your health.

TABLE OF CONTENTS

CHAPTER 1
How I Got Fat and How You Might Too!

If all you care about is losing weight and want to start now, skip to Chapter 7.

Spring of 1995 my grandmother passed away. I packed my bags and headed home to Chicago. I had now lived in the all-you-can-eat three-times-a-day dorm for a year and a half. This trip was going to be an eye opener. My suit, which had not been worn since high school, no longer fit. The jacket barely wrapped around my back and there was no hope of buttoning the pants. The pants were a 32 and I looked like 10 lbs. of @!#$% in a 5 lb. bag. Not good, I had a few hours to be at a wake in a suit.

Off to the mall for a suit. Of course since I had gained so much weight, off the rack suits were not going to work. Jackets were big in the shoulders and tight in the waist. My waist was a round 34/35 and my inseam a 30...this meant a higher end suit and tailoring ($$$$). Fortunately the store offered tailoring and in an hour I had a suit that kind of fit. The 36-inch waist pants were hemmed to a 30 inch inseam and I have no idea what they did to the jacket. I was tipping the scale at over 200 pounds, and still paid no attention to my ballooning weight!

Junior year started in the fall of 1995 and I moved into an apartment. With the move into the apartment I also moved into larger pants. My 34/35 inch pants were boxed and stored to make way for 36-inchers. The good news was that after a semester in another major I was taking a shot at engineering again. A number of my friends helped me with my homework, tutored me when necessary and shared study habits that worked for them. Much to my surprise the denim jean companies had two wonderful new cuts of jeans. I could now get "36 inch Baggy Style" or "36 inch Loose Fitting". Not only did these duds fit but they had plenty of material to grow into. With room to grow I paid even less attention to my weight or eating habits.

1

In the apartment I became a fan of Tombstone and Encore. Tombstone as in pizza and Encore as in "Family Meals." Rip open the plastic or tear the box, crank up the oven, in about a half hour "Let's eat!" Add some instant mashed potatoes, a few pops, and you have a gourmet meal. Grab a plate of food or the whole pizza and off to the living room for an hour or two of TV. Of course there was one added bonus...my roommates liked Tombstone as well but could not eat the whole pizza alone. So I often had an evening snack of their left overs.... usually around the start of my second hour of TV watching.

The weight was still coming on a few pounds a month. With my "Room to Grow" pants, I did not notice. It is amazing how oblivious we are to the gradual and incremental weight gain. Most astonishing is the mind's ability to convince, you that you really have not gained that much weight. The mind can come up with a myriad of reasons for the need to get bigger clothes, none of which included the realization that I was getting FAT.

Spring of 1996 and I was tipping the scales at over 230 lbs. On my 5'7" frame it should have been obvious, but of course it wasn't. My loose or baggy fit 36" jeans and elastic waist warm up pants concealed what was going on. Reality was about to set in. Spring meant interview time. Since I had cleaned up my grades and was in the Mechanical Engineering program it was time to find an engineering internship.

I had the grades, a great resume, and my high dollar tailored suit. I was ready. Line up the interviews then pick the right job for me. The garment bag containing my suit was dug out of my closet to have the suit dry-cleaned and starched nice and crisp. For some reason, maybe the money it cost, I decided to try it on. The pants pulled up to my waist. All progress came to a screeching halt there. The pants would not button. No way...these pants were a 36 and fit great less than a year before.

Not anymore. The "suck in the gut" and button the pants game was played for a few minutes. No go. The pants no longer fit. Reality check. My waist was over 6 inches larger than my inseam. Reality check, how am I going to interview for jobs without a suit. Reality check, I do not have a few hundred bucks to buy a new suit. Panic. Wow! I have gotten Fat! When did this happen?

I finally realized my weight gain. Gradual changes that had gone un-recognized were now crystal clear. In less than 3 years my weight shot from 165 to 230 lbs. plus. My waist grew from 31/32 to a tight 36. This was a watershed moment for me. Unbeknownst at the time, most overweight people that seek change eventually have one of these moments. Their own wakeup call and realization they have gained weight. I was Fat. I now knew it and something had to change. Change should be simple. Just like with grades and school. The same steps I used to fix my grades would work for fat loss.

- Set a goal
- Find someone that has already done it
- Create a plan
- Execute your plan and work towards your goal

Fat loss should be easy. The goal was set, lose weight. On to step Two. Find someone that had done it. This proved to be quite difficult. I was quick to learn two things. First there are plenty of clever marketing people eager to take your money on fat loss gimmicks. Second, many of the so called "experts" (even those with degrees) had never experienced what I did, being fat. The experts were body beautiful people that had no clue what it was like to wake up one day and realize they were fat. They had never been fat!

I tried the fat loss miracle diets and training programs. Even worse were the recommendations of the experts. Here is this body beautiful dietician telling me to do cardio and eat less fat. Gee thanks, I have been doing that and I am not losing weight. The answer, "oh, eat less calories and do more cardio." My experience was screaming these people personally had no clue what it took to lose weight. It was like they went through life fit appearing, felt bad for people that weren't, and pursued a career to help those that were overweight.

It was soon evident that if I wanted to change I was going to have to go it alone. No role models. My pursuit for fat loss led to personal education. Book after book was read. Seek out those that knew what it was like to be overweight, make the decision to change and see that change through.

The result? I have maintained a bodyweight of 175 lbs. at 10% body fat for over a decade. My 36 inch waist is now 30 inches most of the year. My first hand experience became the impetus for a personal training and fitness consulting business and eventual purchase of a health club. Through my business my methods have been used to help hundreds of people of all walks of life lose fat and keep it off .

Personally, I have walked the walk. I have been fat and tried everything and today I know what works for most people. With confidence I say most people because I have helped others do the same thing.

CHAPTER 2
Food, What Is It and Are We What We Eat?

Certainly we are not literally what we eat. If it were there would be Hamburgers, Fries and Pizzas walking among us, though there is some truth to the statement. If we overeat and consume a diet high in "junk" foods we will end up unhealthy and fat. In fact overeating junk food greatly increases the likelihood of weight gain.

So what makes up our food? Macronutrients - Carbohydrates, Fats, and Proteins. There are 3 essential fatty acids and 8 essential amino acids. Essential means we must eat them in our diet. Fatty acids come from fats and amino acids are found in proteins. Interestingly, there are NO essential carbohydrates.

Carbohydrates (Carbs):
Carbs are the body's preferred source of energy. The body begins digesting them in the mouth and can quickly convert the carbohydrates to glucose for immediate energy usage, liver glycogen replacement, and/or storage in muscle and the excess as fat for future use. The carbohydrates stored in the muscle are glycogen and are the fuel that we burn during weight training workouts.

Carbs are NOT essential, but we do need SOME! The key word is SOME, and many overeat them. (1)

Fat
In recent years fat has been the macronutrient bad guy responsible for growing waistlines and increasing heart disease. This is true to an extent. To an extent is the key word. Why? Fat contains 9 calories per gram, over twice the calories per gram as protein and cabs (this will be discussed again a bit later).

10g Fat	90 Calories
10g Carb	40 Calories
10g Protein	40 Calories

Over consumption of fat can be a problem and contribute to weight gain. But, the greater problem lies in the type of fats most people consume and over consume. Yes you read that right. All fats are not the same. There are three types of fats:

Saturated fats: Fats in this category come from meat, dairy, and poultry. When these fats are at room temperature or colder they are solids. At elevated temperatures they become liquid. Over consumption of these fats can aggravate or create the negative health effects associated with fat consumption, namely heart disease.

Trans-fatty acid: These fats do occur in nature, which means we manufacture them. The bubbling of hydrogen through vegetable oils creates trans-fatty acids (sometimes this type of fat may be listed as hydrogenated oils on an ingredient label). Two of the most common applications of this are the making of peanut butter (not the natural varieties) and margarine. The process allows the final product to remain semi-solid at room temperature and can extend the shelf life of a product. There are many other processed foods that have high amounts of trans-fatty acids (hydrogenated oils). There is a strong correlation between negative health implications (especially heart disease) and the consumption or over consumption of these fats. These fats should be consumed sparingly and ideally completely avoided.

Unsaturated fats: Usually found in vegetables, seeds and nuts. In this category there are two important classifications. The essential fatty acids (EFAs) are fats that the body requires and which cannot be made from other fats. They must come from the diet. Fish, olive and flax seed oil are examples of rich sources of these EFA's.

Fats serve a number of roles in the body from hormone production to healthy hair and skin. The good fats (EFAs) can reduce the bad cholesterol (by increasing the good cholesterol or HDL), increase metabolism, reduce joint pain, and more. Fats also increase satiety from a meal by slowing the digestion process down. This means you stay full longer. Most importantly eating fat does not make one fat. So fats should definitely be a part of one's diet, emphasis should be placed on the unsaturated fats especially the EFAs. Can you survive without eating fat? To some degree. But overall health can best be achieved by eating some fat.

Protein
Protein like carbs has 4 calories per gram. Protein is comprised of amino acids. Amino acids are responsible for the repair of lean tissue. For this reason protein is KING. Consider building a house, Protein is the Lumber! No lumber no house...in the case of the human body, no protein no tissue repair or growth.

Protein is made of different amino acids. For simplicities sake we will not cover all of them. There are essential and non–essential amino acids. **Essential Amino Acids must be consumed from our daily diet!**

Proteins are most often found in meats, dairy products, poultry, and nutritional supplements. Since there are different amino acids, and different foods contain varying amounts of some or all of the amino acids, not all proteins are equal.

Though protein is primarily used for the repair and growth of tissue it can also be used for energy. This is especially true when on a low carb diet. In this state the body is forced to look for alternative sources of energy. The body can convert protein to glucose, albeit very inefficiently. For our purposes this simply means that if you eat 10 grams of protein all 10 grams cannot be converted to provide 10 grams of glucose, and it costs calories to do this.

Calories
What is a calorie or kilocalorie (kcal) which is the proper term? A calorie is the amount of heat required to raise 1kg of water 1 degree Celsius. Muscles produce heat when they work. The amount of heat is measured in calories. In the world of health, fitness and fat loss this is important as calories are used to measure energy. Carbs and protein provide 4 calories per gram, while fats contain 9 calories per gram. From this it can be seen that fats provide more energy per gram than either carbs or proteins.

Each of the macronutrients exerts a different effect on the human body when consumed. For this reason, all calories are not created equal if we look beyond calories as a measure of energy. The impact of the calories on the body matter as much as the total number of calories consumed. To illustrate let's take a look at carbs. Carbs create elevated levels of blood sugar. This elevated blood sugar leads to an increase in insulin production. The greater the carbohydrate intake, the larger the insulin response and the harder it is to burn fat.

Different carbohydrates create a different insulin response. This is determined by the glycemic index (GI) of the carbohydrate. Carbs that have a higher fiber content (whole grains) will have a lower GI than those that have little to no fiber (white bread). The higher the glycemic index the faster the carb is converted to blood sugar and the greater the insulin response. Insulin is a storage hormone and when it is elevated it is hard for the body to burn fat.

Fats and proteins can slow the digestion and absorption of carbohydrates regardless of GI, potentially reducing the insulin response. Anecdotally, many have reported to the author having an easier time watching what they eat and they are fuller longer when eating greater amounts of proteins and fats. Empirical evidence and research has begun to show that there may be some validity to this. Some research has indicated that satiety (2), being full, is common in diets higher in protein and fat.

Notes:
There are Essential Fats and Amino Acids (Protein) so they MUST be consumed in our daily diet. Eating Fat will not make you Fat! All Calories are not equal when we they are seen as more than just a measure of energy (3) Glycemic Index is just as important as calories.

CHAPTER 3
Insulin, the Most Powerful Drug In the World, and It's Making You FAT!

Insulin:
Insulin is a storage hormone. In a generic sense insulin can be seen as a school bus that transports nutrients to the different tissues of the body. This makes insulin very necessary to our existence. Though necessary, the continual elevation of blood sugar and insulin can lead to insulin resistance. This roller coaster effect across a lifetime can lead to insulin dependence via prescription pill or injection. This is called Type II or Adult onset diabetes. Type II diabetes is often the result of lifestyle (4).

In addition, when insulin levels are elevated the body cannot easily burn fat due to the hormonal relationship between insulin and hormone glucagon. So we have an inversely proportional relationship of the following: insulin levels up, (glucagon down) fat burning down and insulin levels down (glucagon up) fat burning up. Real simple, when insulin is elevated, glucagon is down, and fat burning is down. If we lower or control insulin and in doing so raise glucagon more fat is burned (5)!

It is like a children's teeter totter. On one end is insulin, the other glucagon. When the insulin side of the teeter totter goes up, the glucagon side goes down. **When insulin is elevated (from lots of simple carbs or sugar) you cannot burn fat!** Here are some other problems fluctuating blood sugar levels may contribute to

- Depression
- Mood Swings
- Sweet Tooth**
- Food Cravings/Addiction **
- ADD/ADHD
- Lack of Energy
- Binge Eating

**Carbs are Addictive and may Cause a "Sweet Tooth"

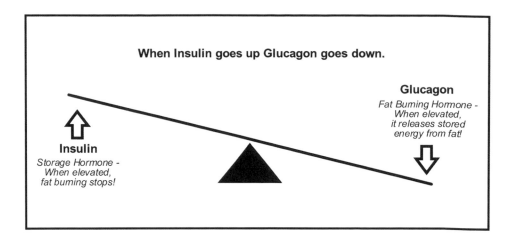

The sudden rise and fall of blood sugar tells the body to eat more. Not just eat more, but more foods with a high glycemic index which will rapidly raise blood sugar again. Pretty easy to see why some individuals have a sweet tooth, an addiction to junk food.

Steady insulin levels will do more than help you lose fat. They will help you feel better in almost every aspect of your life. Stable insulin levels are key to long-term fat loss and health. Stable insulin levels will allow the body to metabolize stored body fat and may reduce the risk of diabetes later in life.

Notes:
Elevated insulin will prevent or slow the metabolism of body fat.
Insulin is a storage hormone, when elevated it will increase the number of calories stored as fat. The roller coaster up and down of insulin levels can lead to diabetes...AND is no doubt part of the reason for the increase in the diabetic rate in the U.S.

CHAPTER 4
Eat Often and Lose Fat!

Are you eating enough to lose fat?

Sounds strange until you have seen or experienced it, but true nonetheless. It is possible to NOT eat enough to lose weight. Here is how this works. The body is built to survive. If calories are constantly reduced lower and lower the body thinks it is starving. Sensing famine, the body goes into storage mode. Now no matter how little is being eaten, the body still stores the incoming calories as fat. This is the problem with any of the diets that require the dieter to constantly reduce calories. Instead of your metabolism increasing, metabolism grinds to a halt. Research has suggested that eating less than 1000 calories will lower metabolism for most people (6).

This is why diets fail and people end up Yo-Yo dieting. As calories are lowered to lose weight, your metabolism slows down and adjusts to the new amount of calories being consumed. Calories are lowered again and the cycle repeats. At some point the dieter is starving and goes back to eating an amount of calories that used to allow them to lose weight, now it causes weight gain. Increasing the metabolism should be the long-term goal. Instead of telling the body a famine is around the corner, tell the body a feast is coming. Turn the body into a calorie-burning furnace. This is done two ways: by eating and by exercising (this will be covered later.)

Notes:
Not eating enough can stall or stop fat loss.
Dropping calories too low can lower metabolism.

Eat Small Meals More Often
One of the easiest ways to rev up your metabolism is to eat more often. Ditch the three squares a day and shoot for 4-6 meals. These should be small meals.

By eating every 2-4 hours the body begins to sense more food is coming. It thinks feast and not famine. The body is happy to burn body fat when it knows another meal is right around the corner. The body burns calories just digesting food. More meals mean more digestion and more calories burned. This is referred to as "The Thermal Effect of Food."

Notes:
Eating small, frequent meals increases your metabolism.

Do not eat in front of the TV
Do not make the mistake of eating in front of the TV. It is easy to overeat when you sit in front of the TV for dinner. Enjoy the conversation and company of family or friends, but leave the TV off during dinner. I made the mistake of eating in front of the TV. If my program was still on, I kept eating. Pretty soon the whole pizza was gone.

Notes:
It is easy to over eat when you eat in front of the TV.

Thermal Effect of Food:
The thermal effect of food means that your body burns calories to digest it. This is important to the individual interested in fat loss. Carbohydrates are easily digested and have a very low thermal effect. Vegetables on the other hand have a high thermal effect and can be considered to be thermogenic. Your body burns calories to digest them.

This is also true of proteins. The body burns calories to digest protein. The thermic/ thermal effect of food is important because this means that you can eat more of some foods than others and have a lower caloric deficit. So a diet high in protein, moderate in good fats, and low in carbs (starchy carbs not vegetables) can be higher in calories than its high carb, moderate protein, and moderate fat counterpart.

Example
A person eats a 2000-calorie per day diet to maintain weight.

Option A	Option B
2000 Calories	2000 Calories
65% Carb	50% Protein
20% Protein	30% Carb
15% Fat	20% Fat

The individual is likely to see a weight loss in option B for two reasons, stable insulin levels, the thermic effect of food, increased satiety, able to stick with the eating plan.

Notes:
More calories are spent digesting protein and vegetables than carbs or fats.

Thermodynamics and weight loss:
There are rules that govern the world we live in. Take gravity for example. What goes up must come down. Gravity holds us to the earth and keeps us from floating off to the heavens. There are also rules that govern weight loss and weight gain. In the world of weight loss, thermodynamics governs our weight loss or gain. In thermodynamics the Law of Conservation of Energy tells us that we cannot create or destroy energy. In the case of weight loss we are concerned with heat or calories. 'Energy in' must equal 'energy out,' if it does not we have the following two situations:

Weight Loss (diet)
Spend more energy (exercise more, thermal effect of food) than you consume (eat) and the body will burn stored fat to provide the energy needed to perform the exercise.

Weight Gain (over eat)
Spend less energy (exercise less, ignore the thermal effect of food) than you consume (eat) and you will store the extra energy somewhere as fat.

Notes:
Once insulin has been controlled as discussed in Chapter 3 weight loss will be a matter of energy in must equal energy out. This is LAW and cannot be changed. We can work with it or against it, but cannot change it.

CHAPTER 5
Another Fad Diet to Help You Pack On the Pounds

Fad Diets, Why you have Failed on Them:

It seems like every day a new Fad diet or approach to nutrition hits the market. All promise a miraculous fat loss overnight. Few mention exercise and its importance to fat loss. None mention long-term success. The advertisements are appealing and it would be nice to lose fat by taking some magic pill or potion. The fact of the matter is that this is not possible. PERIOD. The good news is that there is some useful information in these diets.

Zero Carb Diets
The most popular of the low carb diets is based on a high fat, moderate protein, and low carbohydrate approach to nutrition. Things like bacon and whole eggs are staples of the diet. Absent are breads, cereals, fruit and every other starchy or complex carbohydrate. With an absence of carbohydrates there is a significant initial loss of weight. Now that is weight, not fat.

When carbs are restricted or removed from a diet a person will lose weight quickly. Unfortunately this weight tends to come more from water than anything else. Though this is not a loss in fat it does do something for the enthusiasm of the dieter, which encourages them to continue.

Zero carb diets would have you believe that you can eat as much as you want. Not true. Eating as much as you want is definitely a marketing ploy. One that grabs you, the dieter's attention. Whether this is good or bad is hard to say. What can be said is the fact that as soon as limitations and restrictions are imposed on a person they are set up for failure. Most diets set limits on calories or the number of points per meal or day. Here is a diet that lifts, or appears to lift , that restriction.

The thermic effect of fats and proteins also allow the dieter to eat more. This is again due to the number of calories spent digesting the fat and protein. Some feel that an individual can eat in the range of 10-20% more calories and still lose weight in comparison to the typical high carb and low fat diets. This means more food can be consumed and removes the feeling of having to limit yourself at mealtime. Again eating more does much for the psyche of the dieter and avoids placing yet another restriction on him or her.

Just as there are good points to this approach, there are some that can be improved upon. One of the areas is the overdependence on fat. As discussed previously, there are different kinds of fat and some are better than others. Unfortunately this diet typically relies on the bad fats, the saturated fats found in meats and dairy products. The fats that have been associated with increased potential for disease, most specifically heart disease. Individuals wishing to try this diet need to be aware of this and place a greater emphasis on the good fats.

A second area of concern is the potential lack of fiber in the diet (7). A diet high in good carbs is often high in fiber. When carbs are reduced the amount of fiber consumed is also reduced. Fiber helps control cholesterol and also helps maintain regular bowel movements.

Individuals on this type of diet should make sure to eat non-starchy vegetables (the carbs in them have a negligible impact on insulin levels and will not reduce the effectiveness of the diet). Doing so will increase the amount of fiber consumed and provide additional vitamins and minerals. The addition of a fiber supplement is a good idea as well. The supplement will add daily fiber and also keep the dieter regular. Irregularity has been associated with an increased risk for colon cancer and hemorrhoids. If you are not sure of food sources of fiber or supplemental types, look it up on the internet.

Carbs readily provide the glycogen stored in muscle. This form of stored carbohydrate is what provides the energy for weight training and other forms of anaerobic exercise. Elimination or reduction of carbs, as in a low carb diet, can lead to a lack of energy to perform daily exercise. Longterm fat loss and health improvements require some type of exercise. In order to exercise it becomes necessary to add carbs into the diet somewhere.

Notes:
Some carbs are necessary to fuel workouts.
Cutting carbs completely is a bad idea.
Plenty of vegetables should be consumed daily.
Higher fat meats should not be the staple of daily nutrition.
Cutting carbs cuts fiber, make sure you get 20-30 grams of fiber per day.
Google foods high in fiber and add the ones you like to your daily diet.

High carb, low protein, low fat

The method most commonly recommended for fat loss and health is a diet high in carbs. The food pyramid is often the cornerstone of this type of diet. The high carb, low fat approach to nutrition is high in carbs. Since dietary fat is kept at a minimum the risk for heart disease is reduced, or so proponents of the diet have claimed. If this approach worked so well the rates of obesity and diabetes would not have almost tripled since the 1970s.

Increase In Obesity and Adolescents

Year	Boys Age 6-11	Girls Age 6-11	Boys Age 12-19	Girls Age 12-19
1971-1974	4.30%	3.60%	6.10%	6.20%
1988-1994	11.60%	11%	11.30%	9.70%
1999-2000	16%	14.50%	15.50%	15.50%

Source: CDC, National Center for Health Sciences, National Health and Nutrition Examination Survey. Ogden et al. JAMA.2002; 288: 1727-1732.

Author's Note: If obesity is genetic, were family lines genetically less obese before the 1980s??? Yes, genetics play a role in obesity, but the chart above clearly indicates something else is going on. Statistically, if genetics are the reason we are overweight, where are all of the overweight relatives of the one in three kids born after 2000? Open the family photo albums, where are all of the overweight relatives? **Reality, WE are making ourselves obese and with it unhealthy, WE are responsible for the increase in obesity rate!

Since the high carb and low fat approach is over reliant on the starchy carbs there is a dramatic impact on blood sugar and insulin. The dieter often finds himself or herself hungry and with mood swings. This leads to more carbs and another increase in insulin and blood sugar.

The rise and fall of insulin is what is responsible for that sudden lethargic feeling. That lethargic feeling is often experienced in the morning shortly after breakfast or right after lunch. The problem with the afternoon crash is that the dieter will often reach for coffee, pop, and more simple carbs.

The roller coaster like elevation and then decrease in insulin levels common on a higher carbohydrate diet can spell disaster. Sudden drops in blood sugar result and the dieter often feels lethargic and sleepy after a high carbohydrate meal. Changes in energy levels are not the worst of it either. Fluctuations in insulin and blood sugar can overtime lead to diabetes. Diabetes is the number 3 cause of death and is one that may be prevented through proper nutrition and exercise.

Carbohydrates are not bad. The problem lies in the amount and type that are consumed. How many times have you ordered spaghetti in a restaurant only to have the waitress/waiter bring out what appears to be a bucket of pasta? The same is true of bagels. When was the last time you purchased a bagel in a deli and it did not resemble a Frisbee? Clearly in each of these cases the customer is given a quantity of carbs much greater than a healthy serving.

The production and processing of food has been streamlined and made more efficient. Just as this improves the bottom line of the company producing the food, it increases the waistline of the consumer. Increases in production efficiency necessitate the need for refined, greatly processed and inexpensive (corn syrup, high fructose corn syrup, etc.) raw materials. Great things for manufacturing, but unfortunately the same is not true for the person consuming such foods. These new found efficiencies often cause increases in insulin much the same as table sugar. Now it does not make sense nor sound healthy to consume table sugar by the spoonful. Why would it be sensible to consume foods that have the same effect on the body as table sugar, in mass quantities no less??

The low fat and high carb approach to nutrition for fat loss and overall health does have its good points. Those that advocate this method of eating cannot be faulted. On the outside it looks heart healthy. Reducing the amount of saturated fat (the unhealthy fat) in your daily diet is a great idea. This reduces the risk of heart disease and many other things. Eating fresh fruits and vegetables daily provides essential vitamins, minerals and agents that may help fight or prevent cancer. Again a great idea. But the effect of carbs on the body and its systems cannot be ignored.

Notes:
High Carb and low fat often means feeling hungry.
Over consumption of high glycemic carbs can have long-term health implications (8).
If this method worked so well why has the rate of obesity in the United States tripled since the 1970s?

Calorie Counting, Points, Deal a Diet, and the rest!
There are a number of diets and meal plans based on tracking your daily food consumption. Some have dieters count calories, others track points, and still others pick a meal from a deck of cards. The goal of this approach to diet is to limit the total amount of food consumed.

From our discussion of Thermodynamics earlier we cannot make nor create energy. In other words energy out must equal energy in. When applied to diet this means that to lose weight an individual must eat less calories than they spend and to gain weight they must eat more than they spend. Pretty simple.

The problem is that many of these diets limit what you can or cannot have. This is the problem with all diets. Telling the dieter you can have this, but not that. As soon as that happens the dieter wants that extra piece of bread or an extra 200 calories and over time the dieter will have that extra food. At this point the diet will have failed.

Limiting what a person can or cannot have is a problem. The bigger problem is that this approach is short term. Each of these programs works for a period of time. The dieter sees the scale go down (again this does not mean fat is being lost, remember changes in body fat are what we want to track) and is happy. Eventually the scale stops moving and it is time for a reduction in calories, points or cards from the deck.

When the scale stops moving down your food portions are reduced. This gets the scale moving down again. Alas, the scale stops yet again. Another reduction and things are back on track. The cycle continues. Eventually the dieter is eating very little yet further reductions do not get the scale moving down.

At this point, either the scale is broken or there is a problem. It is unlikely the scale is broken. The latter is true, there is a problem. The caloric level has dropped so low that the body has begun to think it is starving (7, 9). We are incredible creatures built to survive. As such when the body is given the starvation signal and does the opposite of what we want by storing more fat.

Instead of burning fat the body begins to store fat, as it thinks there is a famine, and burns muscle. The frustrated dieter, having existed on minimal food for weeks, considers herself/himself a failure and binges on all the food they have not been eating. With a healthy metabolism this is a recipe for disaster. For our dieter it is a recipe for disaster times ten. Yo yo dieting has begun and it is not only likely that the dieter will gain back all the weight that was lost but as a bonus an extra five or ten pounds.

The good in this diet is portion control. Each of these types of diets teach the dieter how to determine what is a portion. Learning proper portion and serving size is a great start to developing long term healthy eating habits.

Notes:
Focus is on constantly lowering calories, which can lead to a stop in fat loss.
Does not consider glycemic index.
Teaches portion control.

Have a "SlimQuick" shake for lunch and other liquid meal diets.
One highly marketed approach to dieting is the use of liquid meals in the place of whole food meals. There are a number of companies doing this. Some produce

a product that you drink every day for lunch. Others have you drink a gallon or two of their product instead of eating for a few days. Both claim to provide all the needed vitamins and minerals.

Some claim a dramatic reduction in weight in a very short period of time. This is not hard to believe since for a period of a few days you are not going to eat any food. Additionally, the company does not point out that some of the marvelous ingredients exert a mild diuretic effect. So it is little surprise that in a few days the dieter will lose some weight. Nor is it a surprise that much of this weight loss is from lost water and a lack of food. Drinking only calorie free caffeinated beverages and taking a laxative would probably have the same effect. Drinking coffee and taking laxatives does not make sense so why does drinking a few gallons of some citrus potion?

The drink for lunch approach to nutrition has its problems as well. The products typically contain 200-250 calories. With the average lunch containing many more calories it is easy to see how a person could lose weight with this product. A simple look at the numbers demonstrates this quite clearly.

```
Typical lunch . . . . . . . . . . . . . . . . . . . . . . . . . . . 500 calories
Magic Drink . . . . . . . . . . . . . . . . . . . . . . . . . . . 250 calories
Caloric Reductions . . . . . . . . . . . . . . . . . . . . . .250 calories
Weekly Caloric Reduction . . . . . . . . . . . . . . . .1750 calories
```

Theoretical Fat Loss per Month 2 lbs **
**Based on 3500 calories in one pound of fat

So in one month by having a magic drink for lunch the dieter will theoretically lose a half-pound per week or 2 pounds per month.

At first this looks pretty good and simple. Just a shake a day and lose 2 pounds. How could there be something wrong with this?? A quick look at the ingredients of these products paints an interesting picture. The typical ingredients include sugar, fructose, corn syrup, high fructose corn syrup*, and more. In other words, SUGAR SUGAR SUGAR SUGAR. Nutrition high in SUGAR clearly does not make sense and it shouldn't. Remember it is not just about total calories, but how those calories impact insulin and the body!

*Increased consumption of fructose, corn syrup, high fructose corn syrup, and others is being recognized as a large part of the reason for an increase in obesity (10) and diabetes in the U.S (10, 11).

The positive in this diet is that if meals are convenient they will be eaten. There is nothing wrong with having a quick simple meal. This works well for long-term fat loss.

Those always on the go will find success by looking for simple, quick meals...just not ones loaded with sugar and empty calories.

Notes:
Over reliance on liquid meals can lead to a deficiency in certain vitamins, minerals, and fiber. Many liquid meal plans are liquid sugar. Finding fast, convenient meals is important to long term fat loss and health, just not from sugar loaded drinks.

Diets:
The problem with all diets is that they are diets. Diets are short-term approaches to a long-term problem. Fat loss and health are long-term concerns. Looking to address them with a quick fix is doomed to fail. Eating is a long term necessity to live.

Long-term fat loss and health means entire food groups are not eliminated. It means that things are done to increase the metabolism, not lower it. This means eating more not less. Any approach to nutrition that eliminates entire food groups or sets limits by way of points or calories for the Dieter will fail.

The body is built to survive. Gradually reducing calories as most diets do tells the body it is starving. As a result a few things happen. First the body goes into storage mode and starts to slow the metabolism down. This makes losing body fat difficult if not impossible.

Next the body starts to get rid of muscle. Muscle regulates metabolism. The more muscle you have the faster your metabolism. The less muscle you have the slower your metabolism. Think of muscle as expensive. Instead of the cost being in dollars it is in calories. Fat is not expensive. The body sensing less calories coming in (a smaller pay check) gets rid of the expensive muscle and keeps the fat.

The only long-term solution is to encourage the body to burn calories, not store them. This means one has to eat. Eating the right foods and enough of them is critical. That is the premise behind Eat by Color! With Eat by Color! there is no calorie counting, no elimination of entire food groups, and most importantly no dieting! Just a simple approach to fat loss. Fat loss so simple a child could follow it.

Notes:
Long-term fat loss and health require a long-term approach, not a diet. Maintaining muscle mass and with it metabolism is critical to long term fat loss and health.

CHAPTER 6
Your First Step to Losing Weight

How much Fat do you want to Lose and When?

The first step to success with Eat by Color! is setting a goal. In health and fitness, fat loss and weight gain goals are essential. This is not different from any other area of your life. To be successful you have to have a clear vision of what it is you want. Whether in business, family or traveling you must know exactly what it is you want or where you intend to go. In the case of traveling, if you are on the East Coast and want to go to California, simply heading west is not going to get you there.

The same can be said for losing fat and improving health. Simply stating that you want to "lose weight" or "get more toned" will not get the job done. You have to clearly define what "lose weight" or "get more toned" means. This is a very individual thing. What one person may consider success in losing weight or becoming toned another may not.

Determine exactly what it is you want. Write the goal down and tell everyone. Statistics and history demonstrate those who set goals and write them down are most successful in attaining them. Certainly there is one area of your life where you have been successful. In this case it is probable that there was a clearly defined goal, win the little league championship, be promoted, graduate from high school, etc. At some point this goal was written down and people were informed of your intentions. Draw from this experience!

Telling others is extremely important as well. It is often very easy to break promises that have been made to oneself. Procrastination allows us to put things off and just do it later. However, when that promise is made to others it is much more difficult to stop short. Whether it is fear of ridicule from others for not following through or the sense of letting others down, the bottom line is promises and commitments are much harder to break when made to others. This very fact is often the reason that people are so successful at achieving their goals when working with a personal trainer. Commitments have been made to the trainer, financially and other wise and these commitments serve as an obligation that is often hard to break. The result is attainment of your goal.

Everyone has success in some areas of their life. These successes can serve as a tool in health and fat loss as well. Maybe you are the president of an organization, the best bowler in your league, or you have the cleanest car in town. The bottom line is you are successful at or in something. You weren't born any of those things. You consistently worked at it. Fat loss is no different.

Today we have the ability to shape our lives and most definitely our bodies. If we can influence others to elect us to a position in an organization, control a ball rolling down a bowling alley or keep the car extremely clean regardless of the weather or kids, we can certainly choose the direction of our body. Your body is the one thing that you can really control.

Certainly achievement in other areas of life did not come easy. Nothing does. But at some point you kept getting back up and trying again regardless of the stumbling blocks. Most importantly you probably believed that you could do it. Being healthy and losing weight is no different. It is not always going to be easy. Many self help and improvement books recommend finding a mentor, some one already successful at what you want to do and model them. Who better to model than you? Take the area you are already successful in? What did you do to become successful and how can you do those same things to be successful in losing fat?

Successful people share a common trait. They believe in what they are doing and keep trying. Life throws a curve ball and maybe they strike out. But you can bet they are back up at the plate the next inning to take another swing. Successful people are not necessarily born to be good at whatever it is they do. Weight loss and health are no different. There are going to be setbacks.

You control you!!

You are no more born to be a great bowler than you are to be fat, skinny or unhealthy. Recognize and have the courage to keep getting back up. As long as you keep trying you will succeed.

Notes:
Fat loss and long term health improvements begin with a goal and a plan.
Being successful in losing fat is no different than being successful in other areas of your life. Model your own behavior in other areas of your life where you have been successful.

24

The Eat by Color! color coded simple approach to nutrition:

All of the guesswork has been removed from nutrition. No points, calories counting or entire food group elimination. Just a simple, long-term nutritional approach to fat loss and health.

As the name implies color is used in this approach to nutrion. The food groups have been colorcoded. Insulin and its impact on fat loss was discussed earlier. We are going to control insulin to turn the body into a fat burning machine. Eat by Color! focuses on controlling insulin and in doing so raising glucagon. Remember when we raise glucagon we burn fat for energy. Most importantly the focus is on eating to lose fat! Yes, eating, not dieting, to lose fat.

Proteins (Blue): Group 1
If it was walking, flying or swimming it is protein.
Cottage Cheese
Yogurt
String Cheese
Veggie (Meatless Patties)
Soy
Chicken
Lean Beef
Turkey
Fish
Protein Powder
Eggs
*Lean cuts of red meat often have the same amount of
saturated fast as an equivalent amount of chicken breast.
So lean meat is not that bad for you. Red meat is rich in
iron, zinc and B vitamins; enjoy the occasional red meat.

Non-Starchy Vegetables (Green): Group 2
If you can grow it in your garden it is probably going to fall into this group.

Asparagus
Broccoli
Lettuce
Green Beans
Radishes
Green, Red, Yellow, Orange Peppers
Hot Peppers
Spinach
Tomatoes
Onions
Mushrooms
Cauliflower
Celery
Cucumbers
***You can eat as many or as much of these as you like!
They can be added to meals that do not include them!

Insulin Impacting Fruits (not dried/canned) (Red): Group 3a
Apples, any variety, Granny Smith are best
Bananas
Pineapple
Cantaloupe
Cherries
Grapefruit
Grapes
Honeydew Melon
Nectarines
Oranges
Papaya
Peaches
Plums
Raspberries
Blueberries
Blackberries
Strawberries
Mangos
Watermelon
Pears
Unsweetened frozen fruits are acceptable as part of your total fruit intake.
***Focus on the bold fruits as they are more thermogenic (in a generic sense this means your body has to burn lots of calories to digest them, very cool!) and have a lower sugar content.

Insulin Impacting Carbohydrates (Red): Group 3b

What we traditionally call starches or complex carbs.

Rice, white, brown
Potatoes, sweet, white, red, etc.
Yams
Winter Squash
Pumpkin
Oatmeal
Cous Cous
True Whole Grain Breads
Peas
Corn
Beans and Legumes of all type

***Eat foods from this list sparingly. They are high starch vegetables which easily increase insulin levels. Whole grain breads will have a high fiber content and seem heavy for a loaf of bread when you pick them up. If it does not feel heavy it is not whole grain.

"Healthy" Fats and Oils (Purple): Group 4

Olive Oil
Flax Seed Oil
Fish Oil, EPA/DHA
Sunflower Oil
Safflower Oil
Walnuts
Almonds
Pecans
Cashews
Butter
Heavy Whipping Cream
Flax Meal or Seeds

***Emphasize those in bold. They are rich in the essential fatty acids, or the good fats that promote tissue repair, hormone production, reduce bad cholesterol, raise good cholesterol, maintain elasticity of the skin, improve insulin function, and most importantly these are the fats that are absent from the American diet. Most nuts are acceptable except peanuts, peanuts are legumes, not nuts, and inflammatory for some people.

Free Foods (Black): Group 5

These foods you can eat all you want of.

Spices

Sugar Substitutes, Equal, Splenda, Stevia, Sweet 'n Low

Vinegar

Sugar Free Gum

Unsweetened Coffee and Tea

Diet Beverages

*** The jury is still out on how good, bad or otherwise artificial sweeteners are. Millions of people use them every day with no issue. Buyer beware.

Now you have the food lists in pretty colors, now what?

Notes:

Eat every 2-3 hours you are awake. This speeds the metabolism up. Remember our goal is to increase the metabolism, not slow it down. That is what Diets often do. Now maximize that metabolism increase by eating something from the Blue (Group 1) and Green (Group 2) at every meal, something from one of the Red (Group 3a or 3b) at three meals per day (at least one of these times the food should be from the fruit Group 3a), and something from the Purple (Group 4) twice per day (one of the bold choices as they are rich in the Good Fats). It is that simple.

How to Eat Successfully without Dieting Notes:

Eat Every 2-4 Hours

Eat a Fist Size Serving of Protein at Every Meal (Group 1)

Eat Insulin Impacting Carbs 2 Times per Day (Group 3b)

Eat One Piece of Fruit per day (Group 3a)

Eat 30 Grams of Fiber per Day***

Eat 20-30 Grams of Healthy Fat per Day (Group 4)

Eat all the Vegetables you want as OFTEN as you can! (Group 2)

Drink One to Two Gallons of Water per Day

NEVER ALLOW YOURSELF TO GO HUNGRY

If you really want something, HAVE IT. Life is TOO SHORT.

*** Google it! Want to know sources of fiber? Google "fiber," and pick fiber-rich food sources you like!

CHAPTER 7
Your Eat by Color Plan to Lose Weight

<u>Quick, Portable, and Easy Small Meals</u>

2 Scoops Ultimate Muscle Protein in Water
Light Low Calorie Yogurt, 1-2
String Cheese
Beef Jerky
Handful of English Walnuts, Mixed Nuts, Cashews, Pecans
Turkey Jerky
Venison Jerky
1 Yogurt mixed with 1 Scoop of Protein Powder
Hard Boiled Eggs
Almond Butter and Celery Sticks
Those in bold above are weather proof!

<u>Foods to eat sparingly or outright avoid.</u>
Things to Avoid*

Jelly, Honey, Syrup, Regular Sausage, Juice
Rice, Beans, Lots of Cheese
Get the rice or egg noodles on the side
Get the pasta on the side and ask that they do not bring the bread
The desert table, fried foods, pasta and rice dishes
Mayo, Cheese, Fried Anything
Mashed Potatoes, Biscuits, Corn Muffins,
Bread basket, rice, potatoes, go easy on the salad dressings
Pizza, Bread Sticks, Cheese Sticks

* There are no foods or food groups that should be totally avoided. There are foods that should be eaten sparingly or in reasonable amounts. Save these foods for your free day OR have a fist size portion AFTER you have had your meat, fish or chicken AND vegetables.

Eat by Color! Sample Day

Breakfast
3 Egg whites 2 Whole Eggs
2 Pcs Whole Grain Toast
Peppers, mushrooms, onions
*Make an omelet

Breakfast
Fist Size Blue Group 1
Fist Size Insulin Impacting Red Group 3b
Unlimited Vegetables Group 2

Mid Morning Snack
Protein Shake
*2 scoops equal a fist size serving
12 oz of water

Mid Morning Snack
Fist Size Protein Group 1

1 Gallon of Water per day

Lunch
Chicken breast
Large Salad
Olive oil
*1 Tablespoon
Apple*
*1 piece is a fist size serving

Lunch
Fist Size Group 1
Unlimited Vegetables Group 2
10 Grams Healthy Fat Group 4

Fist Size Insulin Impacting Fruit AND
Piece of Fruit for the Day! Group 3a

Mid Afternoon Snack
Protein Shake
*2 scoops equal a fist size serving
12 oz of water
Strawberries

Mid Afternoon Snack
Fist Size Protein Group 1

1 Gallon of Water per day
Strawberries Group 3a

Dinner
8oz Lean Sirloin Steak
Steamed Asparagus
Fist Size Brown rice

Dinner
Fist Size Protein Group 1
Unlimited Vegetables Group 3
Fist Size Group 3b

Before Bed Snack
Light, Low Calorie Yogurt
*2 scoops equal a fist size serving
12 oz of water
Handful of English Walnuts

Before Bed Snack
Fist Size Protein Group 1
1 Gallon of Water per day
Handful Group 4

The options are endless. Simply look at the Column
on the right and mix and match how you see fit.

Eat at your Favorite Restaurant

There is no reason to fall off the wagon when enjoying a meal at your favorite restaurant. Once in a while it is fine and probably a good idea to have whatever you want and as much of it as you want. Most of the time you should have what you want. On the following page is a way to eat at almost any restaurant with out stopping your fat loss.

Greasy Spoons
2-4 Eggs, omelet's, or Egg Beaters
Cottage Cheese
Fresh Fruit, NOT JUICE
Rye or Whole Grain Toast
Avoid or Eat Sparingly!!
Jelly, Honey, Syrup, Regular Sausage, Juice

Mexican
Large Chicken Breast Salad
Steak, Chicken or Shrimp Fajitas or Tacos
ONE Tortilla, Easy on the Sour Cream and Cheese
All the Vegetables you Want
Avoid or Eat Sparingly!!
Rice, Beans, Lots of Cheese

Chinese
Any Meat, Seafood, Chicken, Beef
Any Vegetables
Avoid or Eat Sparingly!!
Get the rice or egg noodles on the side

Italian
Salad with Chicken
Any meat or fish entrée with Vegetables
Avoid or Eat Sparingly!!
Get the pasta on the side and ask that they do not bring the bread

Pizza Places
Grilled Chicken Salad
Avoid or Eat Sparingly!!
Pizza, Bread Sticks, Beer Nuggets, Cheese Sticks

Fast Food
Grilled Chicken Breast Sandwich
Grilled Chicken Breast Salad
2 Burgers, no Buns
Avoid or Eat Sparingly!!
Mayo, Cheese, Fried Anything

Chicken Restaurants
Broiled Chicken
Grilled Chicken
Salad
Avoid or Eat Sparingly!!
Fried Anything, Mashed Potatoes, Biscuits, Corn Muffins

Steak Houses
Any Steak
Any Seafood
Any Chicken
Salad
Steamed Vegetables
Grilled Vegetables
***Get a double of vegetables instead of the potatoes, bread or rice
Avoid or Eat Sparingly!!
Bread basket, rice, potatoes, go easy on the salad dressings

Fill your Grocery Cart:
Many people starting a life change to lose fat and get healthier are starting from scratch. Eat by Color is easy to follow but if you do not have any of the foods in your house you are dead in the water. One simple tip is to shop the outside aisles of the grocery store. This is where most if not all of the foods to help you lose fat and get healthy. Below is a list of foods that should always be in your freezer, fridge, or pantry.

Author's Note: I have worked with many over the years that had no idea what to buy. After a few clients asked me to go shopping with them I wrote a list to give them so they can shop on their own.

Grocery List

Item	Quantity	Group #
93% Lean Ground Beef Patties	2 lbs.	Group 1
Chicken Breast	2 lbs.	Group 1
99% Lean Turkey Breast	1 lbs.	Group 1
Eggs	2 Dozen	Group 1
New York Strip	2 lbs.	Group 1
Filet	1 lb.	Group 1
Salmon	1 lb.	Group 1
Beef Jerky	4 Bags	Group 1
Light Low Calorie	Yogurt 6	Group 1
String Cheese	1 Package	Group 1
Deli Roast Beef	1 lb.	Group 1
Deli Turkey Breast	1 lb.	Group 1
Grapefruit	4	Group 3a
Frozen Strawberries	2 Bags	Group 3a
Frozen Mixed Berries	2 Bags	Group 3a
Plain Instant Oatmeal	Container	Group 3b
Sweet Potatoes	6	Group 3b
Granny Smith Apples	1 Bag	Group 3a
Rye Bread	Loaf	Group 3b
Whole or Multi Grain Bread	Loaf	Group 3b
Celery	1 Stalk	Group 2
Bag Salad	2	Group 2
Bag Baby Spinach	1	Group 2
Asparagus	1 lb.	Group 2
Red/Green/Yellow Peppers	1 Package	Group 2
Frozen Green Beans	1 Bag	Group 2
Extra Virgin Olive Oil	1 Bottle	Group 4
Peanut Butter	1 Jar	Group 4
Can of Mixed Nuts	Large Can	Group 4
Balsamic Vinegar	1 Bottle	Group 5
Light Low Calorie Dressing	1 Bottle	Group 5
Pure Ground Cinnamon	1 Bottle	Group 5
Equal/Stevia/Splenda/Sweet n Low	1 Box	Group 5

CHAPTER 8
The Secret to Turning the Slowest Metabolism Into a Fat Burning Furnace

No discussion of long term fat loss and health is complete without a discussion of exercise. When it comes to fat loss and health, nutrition is King. Exercise comes in a close second. Exercise can help stabilize blood sugar and with it insulin, lower blood pressure and in terms of fat loss increase muscle mass.

Maintaining or increasing muscle mass is key to long-term fat loss. Remember muscle regulates metabolism. The more muscle you have the faster your metabolism. One pound of muscle raises your metabolism by as much as 35 calories! According to Wayne Westcott , PhD. this is the result of the added muscle mass and the increased energy due to protein turn over by existing muscle as a result of exercise.

This has been stated but is worth stating again. Keep in mind that few people, especially women, will get big and bulky when gaining muscle. The idea of a **woman getting big and bulky from exercise is a very big misconception.** Most men will struggle to gain an appreciable amount of muscle. In fact most women indicate just the opposite happens; they slim down and tone up as they add muscle mass. Even if the scale does not change or goes up, most women will report (and many of my clients have) that their dress size goes down.

A pound is a pound anywhere on earth. So a pound of muscle and a pound of fat both weigh a pound. Muscle is denser than fat. Therefore one pound of muscle is physically SMALLER than one pound of fat.

Example:
If a person loses four pounds of fat and gains 4 pounds of muscle, they are the same weight on the scale. BUT, they are likely to be physically smaller! In addition they have more muscle so guess what, they will burn more calories, even just sitting on the couch watching TV!

To illustrate this remember the following exaggerated comparison

1 lb. of Fat = The Size of a Basketball
1 lb. of Muscle = The Size of a Baseball

Again this is an exaggeration, but you should get the point and it should now stay with you. Also remember that you cannot tone fat!

Notes:
Muscle is denser than fat so it occupies less space.
One pound of muscle is smaller than one pound of fat.
If 3 pounds of fat are lost and 3 pounds of muscle gained, the person weighs the same but is likely to be physically smaller.
Fat cannot be toned!
Muscle burns calories.
Fat does not burn calories.
Gaining muscle increases metabolism.

The Right Kind of Exercise
Exercise is critical to maintaining or increasing muscle, which in turn increases the metabolism. But what type of exercise is best? A combination of weight and cardiovascular training is the best way to exercise for long-term fat loss and health. How often and for how long? 30-60 minutes 4-6 days per week. No more and no less.

Many make the mistake of focusing on cardio. They spend the majority, if not all, of their time on treadmills and elliptical trainers...then ask why they are not losing fat. The answer is simple. Cardio helps burn some extra calories but the real bang for the metabolism buck is weight lifting and building muscle.

Research by Dr. Wayne Westcott and others has demonstrated that inactive adults lose one half pound of muscle every year during their 30s and 40s. For every decade that is a five pound muscle loss. Research by Westcott also points to a gain of 15 lbs. of fat during the same period. This is the result of inactivity and not just being 10 years older. The best way to preserve muscle mass is to train with weights.

Nothing maintains or increases muscle mass like lifting weights. Lifting weights does not mean going to the fanciest health club or becoming a body builder. It simply means you do some type of weight training three times per week for 30-40 minutes. A simple whole body work out is extremely effective and can be done at home with little more than a set of dumbbells and an exercise ball.

Once a point has been made to do some weight training a few days a week cardio can be considered. Weight training is priority number one, when pressed for time always prioritize a weight training workout over cardio.

Like weights nothing fancy is needed to get a fast effective cardio session in. Cardio can be done at home with a pair of gym shoes, a bicycle or even a child's jump rope. It can also be done at a gym or health club on your choice of equipment... anything from stair steppers to spin classes are fair game.

Notes:
Exercise will maintain or increase muscle.
Increased muscle raises your metabolism.
Always do some type of weight training, if there is only time to do weight training OR cardio, not both, choose weight training.

CHAPTER 9
Get Help, How to Hire a Fitness Professional

If you are having a hard time setting up or sticking to an exercise program hire a personal trainer! When you are sick you see a doctor. When April 15 approaches you see an accountant. Why should addressing your exercise be any different? It is no different. Hire a trainer, better yet a Fitness Professional.

When it comes to fat loss, health and fitness - hire a Fitness Professional. A Fitness Professional is more than just a personal trainer. They offer guidance in the gym and outside as well. This information is intended to give you the information you need to find a Fitness Professional that will help you reach your goals.

A true Fitness Professional "Walks the Talk." How so? They eat healthy meals throughout the day, a cup of coffee and some protein bars do not constitute healthy. Meals are planned ahead and time is spent cooking them. A few hours of exercise is part of their weekly routine, week in and week out. No excuses are made for not training. Yes, your fitness professional should be doing these things.

There is an ability to relate. In other words they are not body beautiful. Their level of health and fitness was earned. They weren't blessed with low body fat, a super fast metabolism, the ability to run a 10K, or the strength to lift a mountain. A few times per week they exercise. Fitness Professionals set health and fitness goals for themselves, mark their progress, and achieve them. The goal does not matter, what does is that they set a goal and work towards it. This gives the Fitness Professional first hand perspective to draw from and relate to the client and their goals.

The Fitness Professional realizes that setting goals and holding one accountable is difficult. Whether it is getting up early, or staying up late they find ways to stay on track. Realizing life is always going to throw curves gives them perspective to show you, the client, how to hit the curve ball out of the park.

Often people masquerade as Fitness Professionals but are nothing more than rep counting personal trainers. Many have been gifted with a healthy appearing and toned body. They are "BODY BEAUTIFUL." Yet their lifestyle is anything but healthy. They do not "Walk the Talk." Eating good food every few hours is unheard of. Setting concrete goals and achieving them is unheard of. No this does not mean they have to body build, run marathons, or power lift...it does mean they should know what it is like to set and achieve health and fitness goals. Individuals like this will count your reps while staring lackadaisically into the mirror or space, on your time and dime.

If you have never seen the person training you exercise and see them live off nutrition bars and shakes in the pro shop question their ability to train you. How can an individual that does not eat right, rarely trains, and doesn't set goals for personal achievement help you? The reality is they can't. How can they take someone somewhere they have never personally been? They can't!

Qualities of a Personal Trainer that is a true Fitness Professional!
- Current Training Certification
- Liability Insurance
- List of current or former clients that you may contact
- A "Walk the Talk" approach to health and fitness!

The right personal trainer can make a big difference in attaining your goals. They can help you create a plan to safely achieve your goals. They should serve as a form of motivation in and out of the gym.

The truth in hiring a trainer - the real value and benefit of hiring a fitness professional. Let's set up two scenarios:

A person joins a gym and A) hires a Fitness Professional B) just gets the membership, albeit for a place full of equipment they have no idea how to use.

Scenario 1: Your 3 year old would not sleep last night so neither did you. The insult to injury is you are watching your in-law's dog and she played the "I am going out in the yard and am not going to come in any time soon." Bottom line, you did not sleep a wink all night. Icing on the cake, it is raining, damp, and cold.

A) You paid a Fitness Professional and set an appointment, so you are going to show up, you got financial skin in the game. Regardless of what happened the night before, you are not missing your appointment. You get your body fat checked and are surprised by how high it is. You set goals and your Fitness Professional takes you through your first workout to help you reach them. You are proud of the fact you actually made it to the gym. Even your spouse is shocked that you made it to the gym.

B) You skipped the trainer, it is raining and cold, your kid was up all night, the dog still won't come in. Plus it is raining. You rollover and get an extra hour of sleep and will workout tomorrow.

Scenario 2: You joined the gym two weeks ago. It is full of all kinds of equipment you have no idea how to use. Plus you have that nagging shoulder injury that flares up every time you golf and you hope it doesn't in the gym.

A) You paid a Fitness Professional. They will show you how to safely use the equipment. This includes doing strength training and some cardio. You are shocked that you have been working out and your shoulder has been fine!

B) You skipped the Fitness Professional. It has been two weeks since you joined the gym and you still have not been back. Alas today is the day, you are up early and are going before work. You see Johnny Gymrat doing something and heck he is pretty big certainly you must do it too. So you do and your shoulder flares up, but worse than when you golf. Johnny Gymrat suggests you do a few more reps and offers to spot you saying "it will loosen the joint up." The next day you cannot even move your arm.

Scenario 3 : It has been four weeks.

A) You hired a Fitness Professional. It is your last week of training with her three times per week. She checks your body, it has gone down, but the scale has not budged. She informs you that you have lost fat and gained muscle. So that is why your dress clothes are fitting better! You have learned how to use most of the equipment in the gym. You feel confident and comfortable going to the gym. In a month you have been to the gym twelve times. It has become a habit, one you are ready to continue on your own. Plus you know who to go to when you have questions or need help.

B) You skipped the Fitness Professional. Your shoulder has been on fire. In the last four weeks you made it to the gym twice before you hurt your shoulder, and one of those times was to sign up for the membership. Since hurting the shoulder you have been there once. You jumped on the bike and then the treadmill for a few minutes, got bored and left . Three times in four weeks. What a waste of money. You have realized you are not all that comfortable with all those fit people. The Johnny Gymrat experience confirmed you are just not cut out to workout, plus you have that bum shoulder. You can walk, run or ride a bike at home and will just start doing it there. So for the next eleven months you make a monthly donation to that terrible place that just isn't for you.

Accountability, someone you are paying to meet you at the gym means you are going to show up at the gym. You now have financial skin in the game and will actually show up. Many have developed a lifestyle and pattern of behavior over the last 10, 20 or 30 years. Hiring a trainer is a great way to force yourself to get in the habit of going to the gym 3 days a week. Do this for a month and you are likely to keep the habit as a lifestyle change.

A good trainer also holds you accountable for your actions in the gym. Most importantly working with a trainer ensures your workouts will be safe and produce the results you want. Spend time and make the best choice by hiring a professional. It will help you get the most out of your exercise. You and your results are that important.

Ask the potential trainer for a list of current and former clients. Contact them and see what they have to say!

*Any results presented here were accomplished by healthy clients following a regular program of exercise and nutrition. Increases in lean muscle mass, improved health and fitness, and a loss of body fat are likely but NOT Guaranteed. **Before beginning any exercise program always consult a physician.** Participation in a regular program of physical activity has been shown to produce positive changes in a number of organ systems. These changes include increased work capacity, improved cardiovascular efficiency, and increased muscular strength, flexibility, power, and endurance.*

Notes:
Hiring a trainer makes exercise safer.
A trainer increases accountability and results.
A trainer increases motivation to loss fat and get healthy.
Always consult a physician before beginning any exercise program.
Check the trainer's credentials and speak to some current and former clients.

CHAPTER 10
Supplements: Snake Oil or the Holy Grail of Weight Loss?

In the last few years supplements have become more and more popular. Supplements once used mostly by bodybuilders and athletes have found their way into the kitchen cabinets of most households. But are they necessary?

Supplements serve three functions. The first is to fill some type of nutritional void. Today's food no longer contains all of the vitamins and minerals that it once did. Taking vitamin and mineral supplements ensures that we get all of our vitamins and minerals. The second purpose is for performance enhancement. Supplements can increase the rate at which fat is lost, muscle is gained, or the recovery of an athlete. The third and most important function is convenience. Using high quality protein powder or meal replacement makes it easy to eat 4-6 protein rich small meals per day.

Take Two of These and Melt Your Fat Away...Do Fat Burners Work?

The market is flooded with fat burning products claiming to melt the fat off . Simply pop a few of these magic pills and the fat disappears. No exercise and no diet. Not the case! Losing fat and improving overall health and well-being requires work not just a pill, Period.

Research led to the development of supplements that do work in the real world. Quality supplements do make good nutrition convenient and results faster to attain. But "Caveat Emptor" or "buyer beware" because there are plenty of supplement companies out to make a quick buck with low quality products. Do your homework before you spend your money on a product or company.

Determine your needs and goals and select supplements accordingly. Understand that if a product is marketed as providing drug like results it is most likely false.

Supplements have come a long way, but not that far. Make sure to learn as much about a supplement company as you can before purchasing their products. What is on the label is not always in the product.

Notes:
Supplements make losing fat and getting healthy a bit more convenient.
Supplements are NOT a substitute for proper nutrition and exercise.
Supplements are not a replacement for food, you still have to eat!
Remember fat loss is long term, supplementing for a short term result will not work.

CHAPTER 11
Measure Progress to Get Results

History-if we fail to study it we are doomed to repeat it. That which is not measured cannot be improved. Track your progress!

You have made big changes. You are following Eat by Color and exercising. Progress needs to be tracked. The scale is one common tool used to track progress. There is a problem with this. The scale measures your weight. It is more than happy to tell you if you have gained weight or lost weight. But it never tells you exactly what that weight is. Is it Fat, Muscle, Water? Measuring a change in body weight is useful. A change in weight is only part of the fat loss picture.

A person can lose fat AND muscle. Yes the scale has gone down, but so has their metabolism. As discussed earlier, muscle regulates metabolism so the loss of muscle is very bad for long-term fat loss. It is possible to be Skinny and Fat. Remember the benefits of a nice physique extend beyond appearance; the risk for all disease is increased by being Fat. Disease does not discriminate between skinny fat or big fat.

Successful long-term fat loss is gaining muscle and losing fat. It is common to see the scale actually go up (or the amount of muscle), if one is on the right track to fat loss. This is a great thing, contrary to what many would say about fat loss. ***Author's Note: Countless times female clients after a month of training will comment that the scale has gone up, yet they are fitting into jeans 2 sizes smaller than when they started.***

There are many ways marketed to track fat loss. Many are gimics that do nothing more than make the companies selling them a lot of money. The holidays are a great time for this.

Before a discussion of some of the more popular gimics, or ugh methods, let's talk body fat. Body fat percentage is the most common way to track progress. The key here is just that, progress. The actual body fat percentage matters very little. It is great for argument's sake but not much else. The best, most accurate forms of body fat measurement have as much as 3% error.

If percentage is not that accurate what is? Actual skin fold measurements taken by skin fold calipers. Skin fold readings are typically used to generate the body fat percentage. Changes in skin fold are a simple way to track a loss or gain of body fat. There are different formulas, 3-site, 4-site, 7-site, and 9-site, to get body fat percentage from the skin folds. Again formula does not matter, change in the skin fold measurements does. The more measurements, the better change can be monitored.

Popular Methods

Tanita/Bio Electrical Impedance*
This one takes the cake for making companies rich and doing nothing to help track fat loss. This method electronically measures fat. The user stands barefoot on a scale or holds two handgrips. The impedance is measured and correlated to a body fat percentage. This method is greatly influenced by hydration and electrolyte (salt, etc) levels. Users will vary in body fat percentage by as much as 5-8% in the same day and sometimes more based on fluid and salt intake alone.

Author's Note: I have personally seen my percentage read over 20% when the caliper method has me at 6% or below. This is pre-bodybuilding contest results, where visually it is obvious 20% via impedance is way off!

Under Water Weighing/Hydrostatic Weighing
Equates water displacement to body fat. Have a pool and the equipment? If so can you exhale all of the air out of your lungs? Can you completely exhale the same amount of air every time you are tested? Few will have access to the equipment so there is little point in discussing it further.

BodPod (Remember Mork and Mindy? The BodPod looks like it was Mork's)
Equates air displacement to body fat. Kind of a modern technology applied to the old gold standard, under water weighing. A fast, accurate, and easy test, the BodPod is not readily available. Some larger fitness clubs have them but not all. Once again Caveat Emptor or buyer beware. Here is why. The Bod Pod calculates body fat by volume of air displacement. Your body hair creates error as there is no way to account for the displacement due to your body hair. So if your club does not have a BodPod, don't worry about it. * Those that may have done the test will recall having to wear a bathing cap, this is why.

Skin Fold Analysis
This is probably the best method as it is most readily available. Calipers for doing the measurement range in price from twenty to a few hundred dollars. Most gyms

will have calipers of one type or another. The better calipers are green, made of metal and are called Lange Calipers. Various charts and equations take the sum of skin folds and produce a body fat percentage. As is stated above the more sites checked the better and the change in the skin fold total is more important than the actual percentage.

Your Clothes

If you do not have access to skin fold calipers or the BodPod. How about your clothes? How do they fit? Jump on the scale once every few weeks. If it has not moved but your clothes are fitting looser, guess what you have lost fat and maintained muscle and possibly even gained muscle. Body fat percentage, who cares? You are on track, keep up the good work!

Notes:

The scale is not an effective way to track progress.
The fit of clothes is a simple way to track fat loss.
In-expensive skin fold calipers are an easy way to track progress; the more sites checked the better.

ABOUT THE AUTHOR

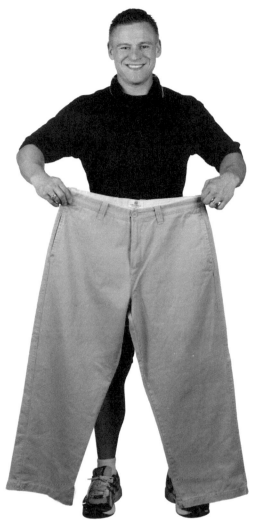

Raymond M. Binkowski

Education:
Bachelor of Science Mechanical
Engineering

Certifications:
American College of Sports Medicine
(ACSM)
Certified Personal Trainer
International Sports Sciences
Association (ISSA)
Certified Fitness Trainer
Nautilus
Certified Nautilus Trainer
Athletic Republic
Level III Master Trainer

Raymond M. Binkowski has personally lost over 50 pounds and kept it off for over 10 years! His waist has gone from 36 inches to 30 (pictured* Ray today behind 36 inch pants.) This first hand experience was paramount in starting a successful personal training business in 2001. In 2007 he purchased a health club and added athletic performance training. Clients include everyday people interested in losing weight. Other clients include professional and world champion athletes, police, fire and military. He has spoken and lectured at colleges, universities, and military bases. Ray is an accomplished author whose articles have appeared in national print and digital media. For more information about Ray and Eat by Color, go to facebook.com/EatbyColor.

REFERENCES

(1) htt p://www.ajcn.org/cgi/content/full/75/5/951-a American Journal of Clinical Nutrition, Vol. 75, No. 5, 951-953, May 2002 © 2002 American Society for Clinical Nutrition[1]

(2)J Am Diet Assoc. 2005 May;105(5 Suppl 1):S24-8.

(3) Nutr Rev. 2009 May;67 Suppl 1:S99-101.

(4) American Journal of Clinical Nutrition, Vol. 80, No. 2, 257-263, August 2004 © 2004 American Society for Clinical Nutrition

(5) American Journal of Clinical Nutrition, Vol. 84, No. 3, 556-560, September 2006 © 2006 American Society for Nutrition

(6) Pretnice AM et al. Physiological responses to slimming. Proceedings of the Nutrition Society (1991) 50: 441-458.

(7) American Journal of Clinical Nutrition, Vol 59, 1242S-1247S, Copyright © 1994 by The American Society for Clinical Nutrition, Inc.

(8) American Journal of Clinical Nutrition, Vol 66, 974S-979S, Copyright © 1997 by The
American Society for Clinical Nutrition, Inc.

(9)American Journal of Clinical Nutrition, Vol 51, 167-172, Copyright © 1990 by The American Society for Clinical Nutrition, Inc.

(10) American Journal of Clinical Nutrition, Vol. 79, No. 4, 537-543, April 2004 © 2004 American Society for Clinical Nutrition

(11) American Journal of Clinical Nutrition, Vol. 79, No. 5, 774-779, May 2004 © 2004 American Society for Clinical Nutrition

APPENDIX A:
Eat on the Go Guide

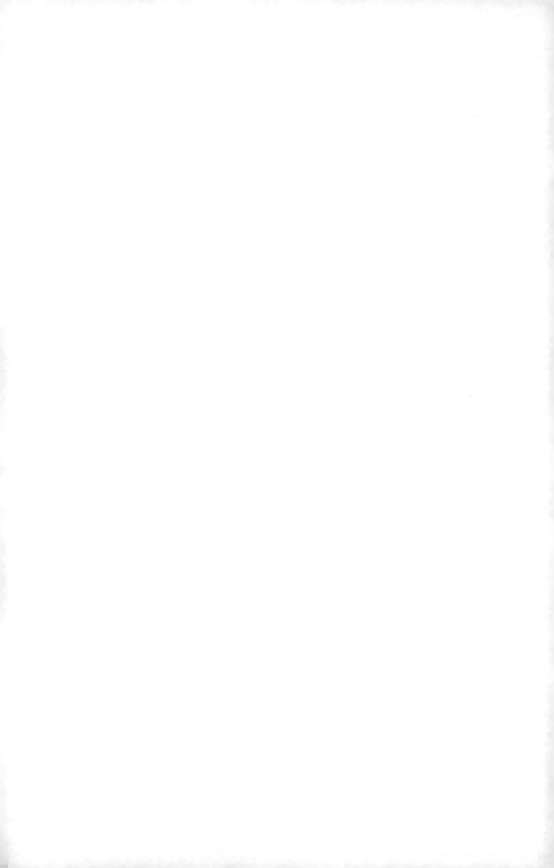

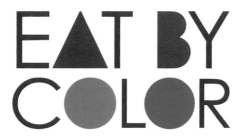

Eat On the Go Guide

How to Eat Successfully without Dieting

Eat Every 2-4 Hours
Eat a Fist Size Serving of Protein at Every Meal
Eat Insulin Impacting Carbs 2-4 Times per Day
Eat One Piece of Fruit per day, Counts for One of 2-4 Above
Eat 30 Grams of Fiber per Day***
Eat 20-30 Grams of Healthy Fat per Day
Eat all the Vegetables you want as OFTEN as you can!
Drink One to Two Gallons of Water per Day
NEVER ALLOW YOURSELF TO GO HUNGRY
If you really want something, HAVE IT. Life is TOO SHORT

*** Google it! Want to know sources of fiber? Google "fiber" and
pick food sources you like!

Eating Out

Greek Style Restaurant
2-4 Eggs, omelettes, or Egg Beaters
Cottage Cheese
Fresh Fruit, NOT JUICE
Rye or Whole Grain Toast
Things to Avoid!!
Jelly, Honey, Syrup,
Regular Sausage, Juice

Mexican
Large Chicken Breast Salad
Steak, Chicken or Shrimp Fajitas or
Tacos ONE Tortilla, Easy on the Sour
Cream and Cheese
All the Vegetables you Want
Things to Avoid!!
Rice, Beans, Lots of Cheese

Asian
Any Meat, Seafood, Chicken, Beef
Any Vegetables
Things to Avoid!!
Get the rice or egg noodles on the side

Italian
Salad with Chicken
Any meat or fish entrée with Vegetables
Things to Avoid!!
Get the pasta on the side and ask that
they do not bring the bread

Buffet
Salad Vegetables
Cooked Vegetables
Lean, Not Fried Meats
Things to Avoid!!
The desert table, fried foods, pasta and
rice dishes

Fast Food, Burger Place
Grilled Chicken Breast Sandwich
Grilled Chicken Breast Salad
2 Burgers, no Buns
Things to Avoid!!
Mayo, Cheese, Fried Anything

Fried Chicken
Broiled Chicken
Grilled Chicken
Salad
Things to Avoid!!
Fried Anything, Mashed Potatoes,
Biscuits, Corn Muffins

Steak House
Any Steak
Any Seafood
Any Chicken
Salad
Steamed Vegetables
Grilled Vegetables
***Get a double of vegetables instead
of the potatoes, bread or rice
Things to Avoid!!
Bread basket, rice, potatoes, go easy
on the salad dressings

Pizza Place
Grilled Chicken Salad
Things to Avoid!!
Pizza, Bread Sticks, Beer Nuggets,
Cheese Sticks

Grocery List

Item	Quantity	Group #
93% Lean Ground Beef Burger Patties	2 lbs	Group 1
Chicken Breast	2 lbs	Group 1
99% Lean Turkey Breast	1 lbs	Group 1
Eggs	2 Dozen	Group 1
New York Strip	2 lbs	Group 1
Filet	1 lb	Group 1
Salmon	1 lb	Group 1
Beef Jerky	4 Bags	Group 1
Light Low Calorie	Yogurt 6	Group 1
String Cheese	1 Package	Group 1
Deli Roast Beef	1 lb	Group 1
Deli Turkey Breast	1 lb	Group 1
Grapefruit	4	Group 2
Frozen Strawberries	2 Bags	Group 2
Frozen Mixed Berries	2 Bags	Group 2
Plain Instant Oatmeal	Large Container	Group 2
Sweet Potatoes	6	Group 2
Granny Smith Apples	1 Bag	Group 2
Rye Bread	Loaf	Group 2
Whole or Multi Grain Bread	Loaf	Group 2
Celery	1 Stalk	Group 3
Bag Salad	2	Group 3
Bag Baby Spinach	1	Group 3
Aspargus	1 lb	Group 3
Red/Green/Yellow Peppers	1 Package	Group 3
Frozen Green Beans	1 Bag	Group 3
Extra Virgin Olive Oil	1 Bottle	Group 4
Peanut Butter	1 Jar	Group 4
Can of Mixed Nuts	Large Can	Group 4
Balsamic Vinegar	1 Bottle	Group 5
Light Low Calorie Dressing	1 Bottle	Group 5
Pure Ground Cinnamon	1 Bottle	Group 5
Equal/Stevia/Splenda/Sweet n Low	1 Box	Group 5

Quick, Portable and Easy Small Meals

2 Scoops Ultimate Muscle Protein in Water
Light Low Calorie Yogurt, 1-2
String Cheese
Beef Jerky
Handful of English Walnuts, Mixed Nuts, Cashews, Pecans
Turkey Jerky
Venison Jerky
1 Yogurt mixed with 1 Scoop of Protein Powder
Hard Boiled Eggs
Almond Butter and Celery Sticks
Those in bold above are weather proof!

Eat Sparingly

Jelly, Honey, Syrup, Regular Sausage, Juice
Rice, Beans, Lots of Cheese
Get the rice or egg noodles on the side
Get the pasta on the side and ask that they do not bring the bread
The desert table, fried foods, pasta and rice dishes
Mayo, Cheese, Fried Anything
Fried Anything, Mashed Potatoes, Biscuits, Corn Muffins
Bread basket, rice, potatoes, go easy on the salad dressings
Pizza, Bread Sticks, Beer Nuggets, Cheese Sticks

There are no foods or food groups that should be totally avoided.
There are foods that should be eaten sparingly or in reasonable amounts.
Save these foods for your free day OR have a fist size portion, no more, no less
AFTER you have had your meat, fish or chicken AND vegetables.

Food List

Proteins: Group 1

If it was walking, flying or swimming it is protein.

Cottage Cheese
Yogurt
String Cheese
Veggie (Meatless Patties)
Soy
Chicken
Lean Beef
Turkey
Fish
Eggs

Non-Starchy Vegetables: Group 2

If you can grow it in your garden it is probably going to fall into this group.

Asparagus
Brocoli
Lettuce
Green Beans
Radishes
Green, Red, Yellow & Orange Peppers
Hot Peppers
Spinach
Tomatos
Onions
Mushrooms
Coliflower
Celery
Carrots

***You can eat as many or as much of these as you like! They can even be added to meals that do not include them!

Insulin Impacting Fruits (not dried or canned): Group 3a

Apples, any variety, Granny Smith are best
Bananas
Pineapple
Cantaloupe
Cherries
Grapefruit
Grapes
Honeydew Melon
Nectarines
Oranges
Papaya
Peaches
Plums
Raspberries
Blueberries
Blackberries
Strawberries
Mangos
Watermelon
Pears   ↓ SUGAR CONTENT

Unsweetened frozen fruits are acceptable as part of your total fruit intake.***Focus on the bold fruits as they are more thermogenic (in a generic sense this means your body has to burn lots of calories to digest them, very cool!) and have a lower sugar content.

2-3 a day

Insulin Impacting Carbohydrates: Group 3b

What we traditionally call starches or complex carbs.

Rice, white, brown
Potatos, sweet, white, red, etc.
Yams
Winter Squash
Pumpkin
Oatmeal
Cous Cous
True Whole Grain Breads
Peas
Corn
Beans and Legumes of all type

***Eat foods from this list sparingly. They are high starch vegetables which easily increase insulin levels.

"Healthy" Fats and Oils: Group 4

Olive Oil
Flax Seed Oil
Fish Oil, EPA/DHA
Sunflower Oil
Safflower Oil
Walnuts
Almonds
Pecans
Cashews
Butter
Flax Meal or Seeds

***Emphasize those in bold. They are rich in the essential fatty acids, or the good fats that promote tissue repair, hormone production, reduce bad cholesterol, raise good cholesterol, maintain elasticity of the skin, improve insulin function, and most importantly these are the fats that are absent from the American diet. Most nuts are acceptable except peanuts, peanuts are legumes, not nuts, and inflammatory for some people.

Free Foods (Black): Group 5

These foods you can eat all you want of.
Spices
Sugar Substitutes, Equal, Splenda, Stevia, Sweet n Low
Vinegar
Sugar Free Gum
Diet Beverages

*** The jury is still out on how good, bad or otherwise artificial sweeteners are. Millions of people use them every day with no issue. Buyer beware.

APPENDIX B:
Bonus Workout Section

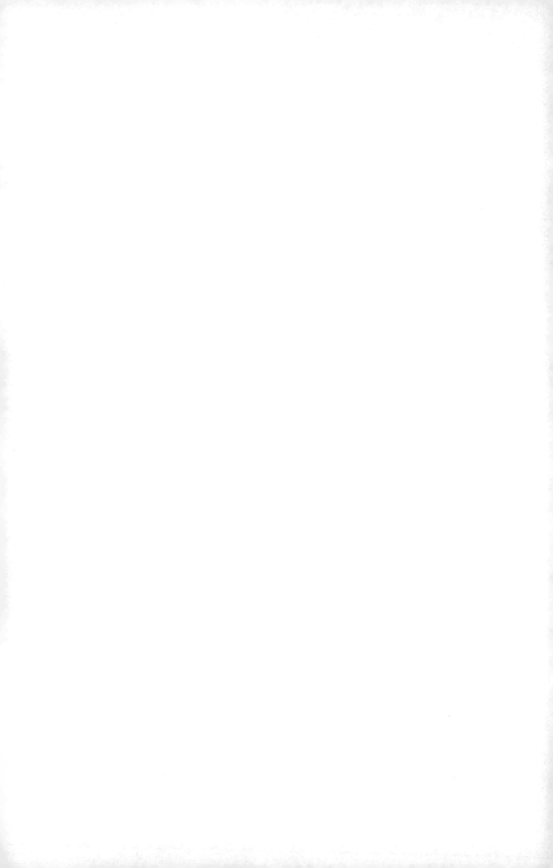

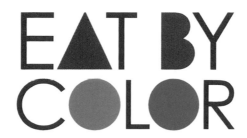

Bonus Workout Section

DISCLAIMER

Raymond M. Binkowski is not a physician or registered dietitian. The contents of this book should not be taken as medical advice. It is not intended to diagnose, treat, cure, or prevent any health problem – nor is it intended to replace the advice of a physician. Always consult your physician or qualified health professional on any matters regarding your health and before beginning any exercise program, including those that follow.

Bonus Workout Section to Get You Started!

The following training programs are intended for healthy individuals free of any type of disease, illness, or injuries. Always consult your physician or qualified health professional before beginning the following or any other training program.

There are three workout programs. Each program should be done for 4-8 weeks. Then go on to the next program. Total workout time per week will be about three hours! Strength train every other day three days per week. Most exercises are done in pairs. So you will do the first set of the first exercise, do not rest (note Rest of 0 seconds) then complete a set of the next exercise, then rest (note Rest 60 seconds.) After strenght training peform the core program.

Three days per week, after strength training, or on the days in between strength training perfrom interval cardio. Each cardio session is only going to take you a total of 20 minutes to complete. Only 20 minutes but you will burn fat at an increased rate for the next 12 to 36 hours. The programs say "Walk, Jog, or Run" but this does NOT mean you have to actually use a treadmill. Each of the programs can be done on a bike, elliptical, rower, stair climber, or treadmill. They can also be done outside.

"Walk, Jog, or Run" are used to describe how hard you are working for that minute. Each minute the intensity will vary. If you have a heart rate monitor and would like to use it you can use your heart rate (FitWorkz sells Polar Heart Rate monitors) instead of "Walk, Jog, or Run." To calculate your theoritical max heart rate subtract your age from 220. Then multiply by 70%, 80%, or 90%. Then use your heart rate to guide how hard you should be working for each of your one minute intervals.

The author thanks the following people for their help with the photos and layout of this guide:
> *Cameron Chenault*
> *Henry Glick*

Program 1

Exercise	Sets	Reps	Rest
Step Up	3	12	0
Single leg squat	3	12	60
Assisted Pull-up	3	10	0
Assisted Dip	3	10	60
DB Bench Press	3	10	0
Db Curl	3	10	60
DB Row	3	10	0
DB Shoulder Press	3	10	60
Core			

CORE

Exercise	Sets	Reps	Rest
Crunch	3	15	0
Bicycle	3	15	0
Toe Touch Crunch	3	15	0
Russian Twist	3	15	0
Plank	3	30 seconds	60

INTERVAL CARDIO

Time	Intensity	HRt
1	Walk	70% Max HRT
2	Walk	70% Max HRT
3	Jog	80% Max HRT
4	Run	90% Max HRT
5	Walk	70% Max HRT
6	Jog	80% Max HRT
7	Run	90% Max HRT
8	Walk	70% Max HRT
9	Jog	80% Max HRT
10	Run	90% Max HRT
11	Walk	70% Max HRT
12	Jog	80% Max HRT
13	Run	90% Max HRT
14	Walk	70% Max HRT
15	Jog	80% Max HRT
16	Run	90% Max HRT
17	Walk	70% Max HRT
18	Jog	80% Max HRT
19	Walk	70% Max HRT
20	Walk	70% Max HRT

Program 2

Exercise	Sets	Reps	Rest
Step Up	3	12	0
Single leg squat	3	12	60
Bosu Squat	3	10	0
DB Squat	3	10	60
DB Stiff Leg Deadlift	3	10	0
Db Curl	3	10	60
Seated Calve Raise	3	10	0
Standing Calve Raise	3	10	60

CORE

Exercise	Sets	Reps	Rest
DB Bench Press	3	12	0
DB Row	3	12	60
Assisted Pullup	3	10	0
Assisted Dip	3	10	60
DB Lying Tricep Ext	3	10	0
Db Curl	3	10	60
DB Lateral Raise	3	10	0
DB Shoulder Press	3	10	60
Core			

Exercise	Sets	Reps	Rest
Crunch	4	15	0
Bicycle	4	15	0
Toe Touch Crunch	4	15	0
Russian Twist	4	15	0
Plank	4	60 seconds	60

INTERVAL CARDIO

Time	Intensity	HRt
1	Walk	70% Max HRT
2	Walk	70% Max HRT
3	Jog	80% Max HRT
4	Run	90% Max HRT
5	Walk	70% Max HRT
6	Jog	80% Max HRT
7	Run	90% Max HRT
8	Walk	70% Max HRT
9	Jog	80% Max HRT
10	Run	90% Max HRT
11	Jog	80% Max HRT
12	Run	90% Max HRT
13	Jog	80% Max HRT
14	Run	90% Max HRT
15	Walk	70% Max HRT
16	Jog	80% Max HRT
17	Run	90% Max HRT
18	Jog	80% Max HRT
19	Walk	70% Max HRT
20	Walk	70% Max HRT

Program 3

Exercise	Sets	Reps	Rest
Step Up	3	12	0
Single leg Squat	3	12	60
Leg Press Wide	3	10	0
Leg Press Narrow	3	10	60
Leg Extension	3	10	0
Leg Curl	3	10	60
Seated Calf Raise	3	10	0
Standing Calf Raise	3	10	60
Core			

Exercise	Sets	Reps	Rest
DB Bench Press	3	12	60
DB Incline Bench Press	3	12	60
DB Fly	3	10	60
DB Lying Tricep Ext	3	10	60
Pushup	3	20	60
DB Shoulder Press	3	10	60
DB Front Raise	3	10	60
Rope Tricep Extension	3	10	60
Core			

Exercise	Sets	Reps	Rest
Lat Pulldown	3	12	60
Seated Row	3	12	60
Close Grip Lat Pulldown	3	10	60
DB Curl	3	10	60
DB Row	3	10	60
DB Hammer Curl	3	10	60
DB Reverse Fly	3	10	60
Core			

CORE

Exercise	Sets	Reps	Rest
Crunch	4	15	0
Bicycle	4	15	0
Toe Touch Crunch	4	15	0
Russian Twist	4	15	0
Plank	4	60 seconds	60

INTERVAL CARDIO

Time	Intensity	HRt
1	Walk	70% Max HRT
2	Walk	70% Max HRT
3	Jog	80% Max HRT
4	Run	90% Max HRT
5	Jog	80% Max HRT
6	Run	90% Max HRT
7	Jog	80% Max HRT
8	Run	90% Max HRT
9	Jog	80% Max HRT
10	Run	90% Max HRT
11	Sprint	All Out
12	Jog	80% Max HRT
13	Run	90% Max HRT
14	Jog	80% Max HRT
15	Run	90% Max HRT
16	Jog	80% Max HRT
17	Run	90% Max HRT
18	Sprint	All Out
19	Walk	70% Max HRT
20	Walk	70% Max HRT

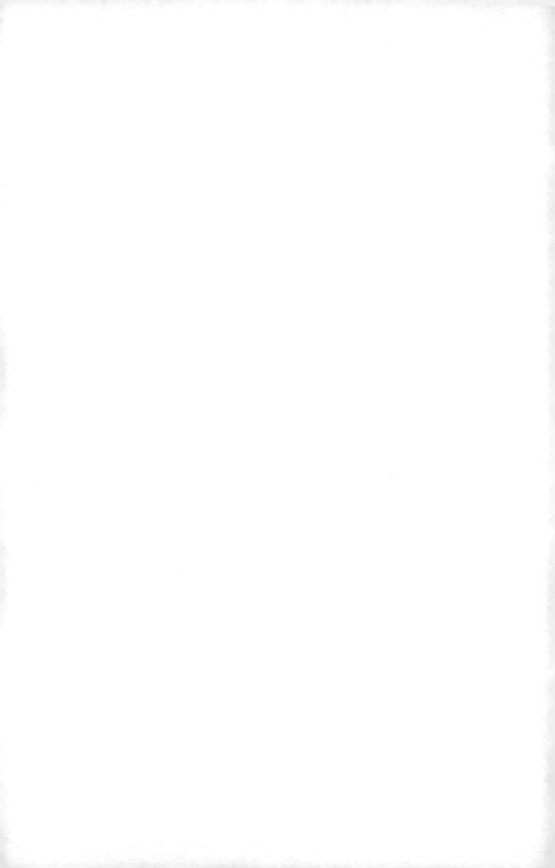

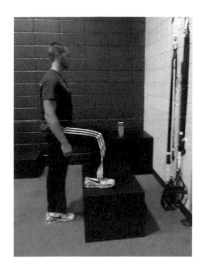 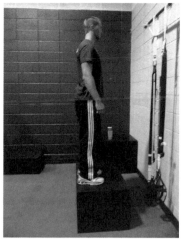

STEP UP
While standing up tall, head up, step onto box with foot facing forward. Step down in the same sequence. That's one rep. Do all reps on one side then repeat.
Works: Quad, Glute, Ham

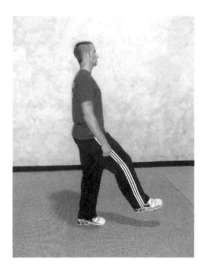 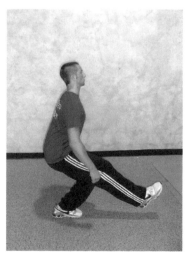

SINGLE LEG SQUAT
While standing up tall, head up, extend one leg in front of you. Bend the oppisite leg and squat as low as you can without falling over. Use arms for balance if needed.
Works: Quad, Glute, Ham

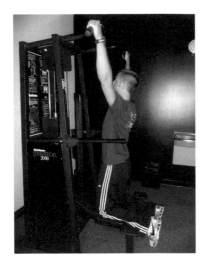 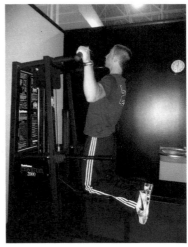

ASSISTED PULL UP

With knees on pad, extend arms all the way out, then pull up until your chin is at the top of the machine. Remember to lift with your back, not your arms. More weight on this machine means it is easier to perform the exercise.

Works: Lats, Biceps

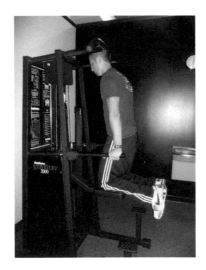 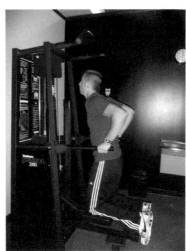

ASSISTED DIP

With knees on pad and hands on dip handles, extend arms all the way out, then bend at the elbow until they are 90 degrees and extend back to starting position.

Works: triceps, chest if leaning forward

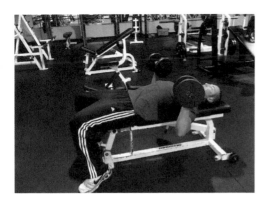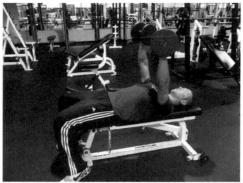

DUMBBELL BENCH PRESS

Start with feet firmly on ground, butt, back and head firmly on bench. With the weights at chest height, extend arms out completely and return to starting position slowly.

Works: Chest, Triceps

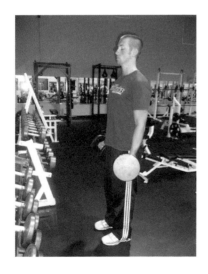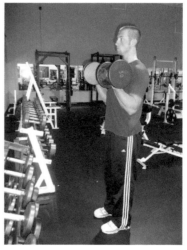

DUMBBELL CURL

While standing up tall, start with weights at sides and curl up with palms facing out. Return to starting position slowly.

Works: Biceps

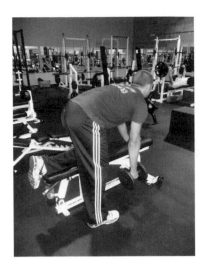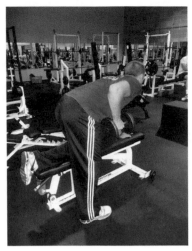

DUMBBELL ROW

Starting with one foot flat on the ground and knee firmly planted on the bench, keep your back flat and head up. With weight dangling at chest height, pull towards your body and back down slowly.

Works: Rhomboids and Middle Trapezius

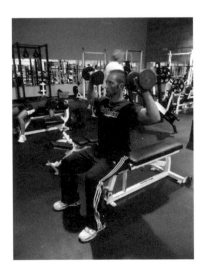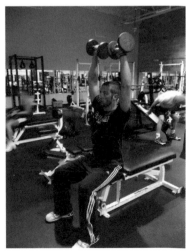

DUMBBELL SHOULDER PRESS

While sitting up tall, weights next to your head as pictured, extend arms overhead and back down slowly.

Works: Deltoids, Trapezius

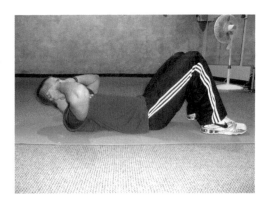 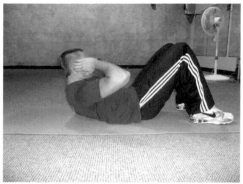

CRUNCH
Start by lying on the ground with feet firmly planted on the ground, knees bent and hands by the side of your head, elbows out. Crunch forward using your abs while trying to bring your elbows toward your knees. Keep neck in neutral spine.
Works: rectus abdominus

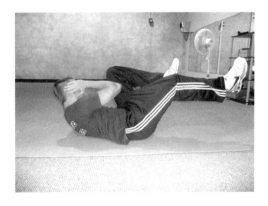 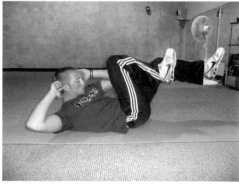

BICYCLE
Start in same position as a crunch but this time elevate the legs. Crunch forward trying to bring one elbow to the opposite knee and alternate back and forth while extending the opposite foot out as far as possible.
Works: Rectus abdominus, oblique

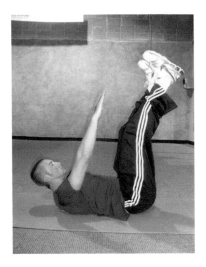 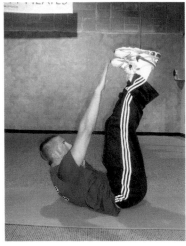

TOE TOUCHES

Start in same position as crunch except legs are vertical over your hips. Perform the exercise while crunching forward, trying to touch your toes. Keep legs straight as possible.
Works: Recuts abdominus

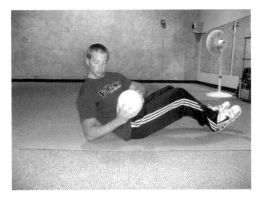 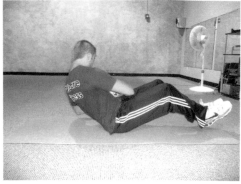

RUSSIAN TWIST

Sit on the ground with heels and butt touching the ground. Hold onto a ball or hold hands together with arms extended. Torso should be at a 45 degree angle with the ground. Twist your torso from side to side. There and back is one rep. To increase difficulty, hold onto a heavier ball and/or raise your feet off the ground.
Works: rectus abdominus, obliques

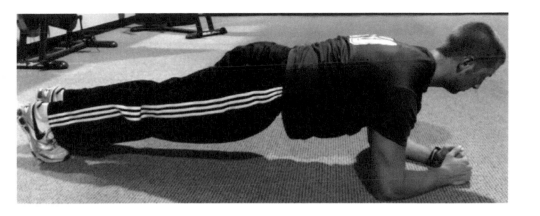

PLANK
Hold the above position for the allotted time. Butt down, back
flat, abs flexed, head and neck in neutral spine.
Works: Core

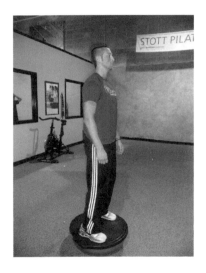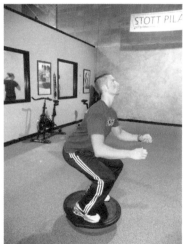

BOSU SQUAT
Stand on an upside down bosu ball. Gain balance before
attempting move. While keeping head up and back flat, bend at
the knees and keep butt back. Bend down to 90 degrees or as
low as possible. Keep arms out in front for balance.
Works: Glutes, Hamstrings, Quads, Core stabilizers

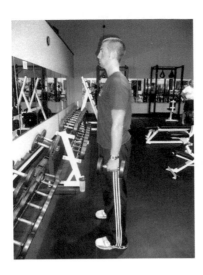 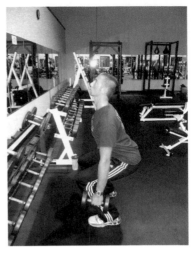

DUMBBELL SQUAT
Start with dumbbells at side, feet shoulder width apart. While keeping head up and back flat, bend at the knees and keep butt back. Bend down to 90 degrees or as low as possible. Keep arms out in front for balance.
Works: Glutes, Hamstrings, Quads

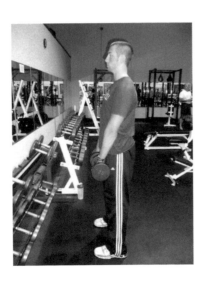 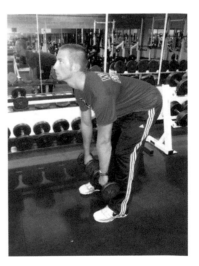

DUMBBELL STIFF LEGGED DEAD LIFT
Start by standing up tall with feet shoulder width apart, weights in front of you. Bend at the waist keeping your head up and back flat. Keeps the legs straight, but knees slightly bent.
Slowly return back to starting position.
Works: Hamstrings

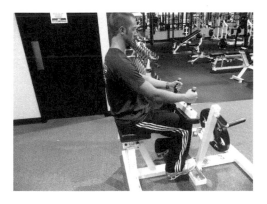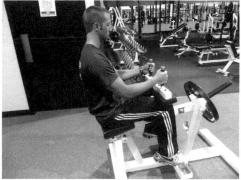

SEATED CALF RAISE
Start with heels below foot bar. Press foot down so the weight
rises as well as your heels move above the bar.
Works: Soleus

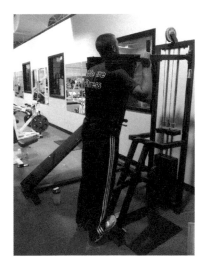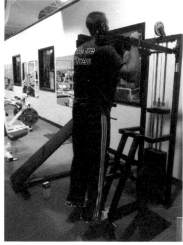

STANDING CALF RAISE
Start with heels below foot bar. Press foot down so the weight
rises as well as your heels move above the bar.
Works: Gastrocnemius

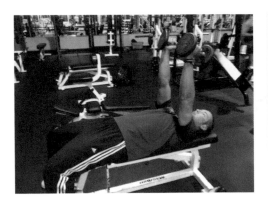 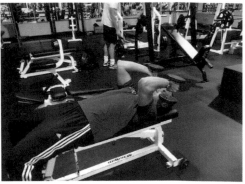

LYING TRICEP EXTENSION

Lying flat on a bench, Raise weight at chest height above you.
Slowly lower the weight down to either side of your head.
Concentrate on keeping the elbows perpendicular to your body
and tucked in, do not let them flare out.

Works: Triceps

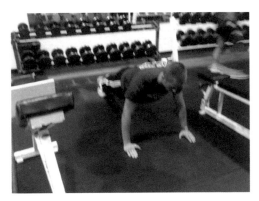 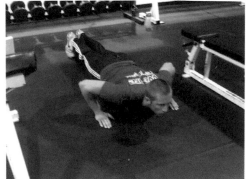

PUSHUP

In a plank position keep head in neutral spine, back flat and butt
down. Lower yourself to the ground so your chest, not your
head or face, is a few inches from the ground.

Works: Chest, Core

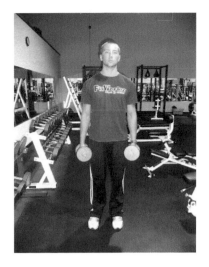 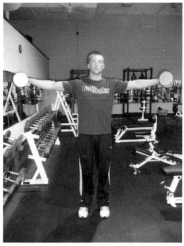

LATERAL RAISE
Start with weight at your sides. Raise the weight out to the side until it is at shoulder height. When performing this exercise try not to swing the weights. Use a lower weight if you need to swing.
Works: Deltoids

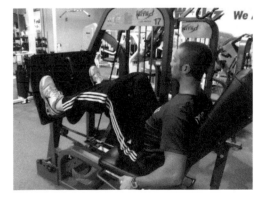 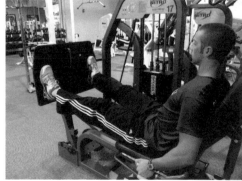

LEG PRESS WIDE
Start with back and butt on the pad. Feet on the plate with toes slightly pointed out. When performing this exercise it is important to first push through you're your heels and not your toes and secondly not to slam your knees into a locked position.
Works: Quads, Hams, Glutes

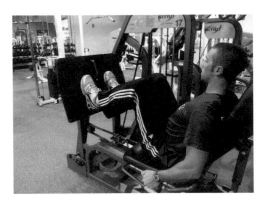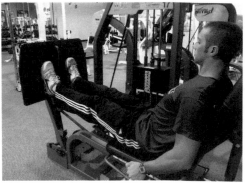

LEG PRESS NARROW

Start with back and butt on the pad. Feet on the plate with toes slightly pointed out. When performing this exercise it is important to first push through you're your heels and not your toes and secondly not to slam your knees into a locked position.

Works: Quads, Hams, Glutes

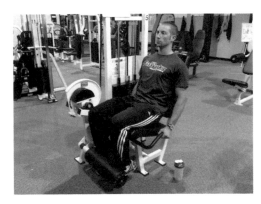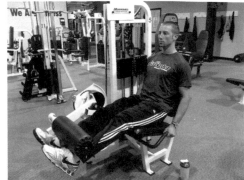

LEG EXTENSION

Start this exercise with butt and back firmly on the pad. Extension pad should be placed at the ankles. Fully extend legs and return to starting position. Use handles to remain seated in the chair.

Works: Quads

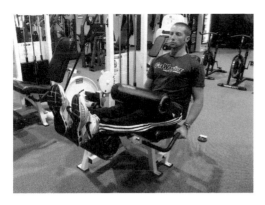 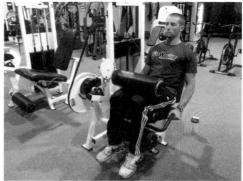

LEG CURL

Start this exercise with butt and back firmly on the pad. Flexion pad should be placed at the back ankles with knee pad just above the knee caps. Fully flex legs and return to starting position. Use handles to remain seated in the chair.

Works: Hamstrings

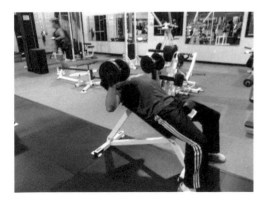 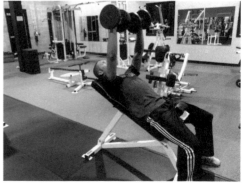

DUMBBELL INCLINE BENCH PRESS

Start with bench at a 45 degree angle and feet firmly on ground, butt, back and head firmly on bench. With the weights at chest height, extend arms out completely and return to starting position slowly.

Works: Upper Chest, Triceps

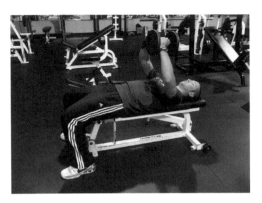
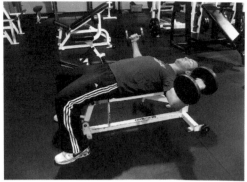

DUMBBELL CHEST FLY
Start with feet firmly on ground, butt, back and head firmly on bench.
With the weights at chest height, keep elbows bent and extend arms
parallel to the floor and return to starting position slowly.
Works: Chest

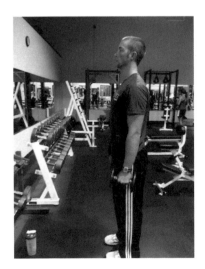
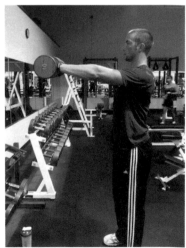

FRONT RAISE
Start with weights in front of you at sides, standing up tall. Raise
weights, palms down, in front of you until shoulder height and
return slowly. Remember not to swing arms.
Works: Front Delts

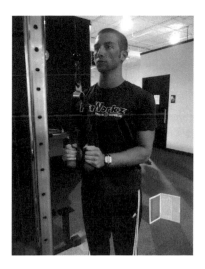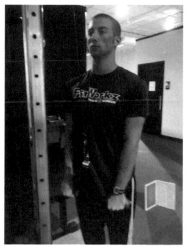

TRICEP ROPE
Standing at a cable cross with tri-rope attached, grab the rope with hands touching the knots or knobs on the rope. Extend arms out and make sure wrists are straight and knobs/knots flare out at the bottom of the movement.
Works: Triceps

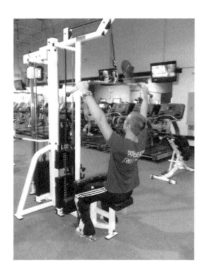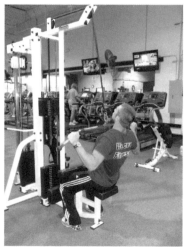

LAT PULL-DOWN
At a lat pull down machine, after setting weight, grab bar with a wide grip and sit down so butt and feet are firmly planted on the seat and ground. Starting with arms extended pull bar towards your chest as far as possible and slowly return to starting position.
Works: Latissimus Dorsi

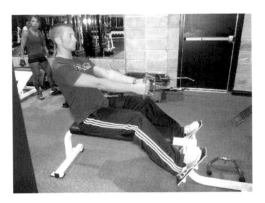
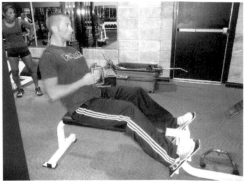

BACK ROW
Make sure butt and feet firmly planted on foot plates and seat.
After setting weight, grab handles and extend legs. Start with
arms extended and pull handle to your chest. Do not bend or
rock at your torso, movement should only occur at the arms.
Works: Rhomboids, Middle Trap

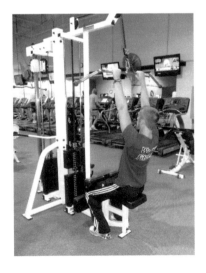
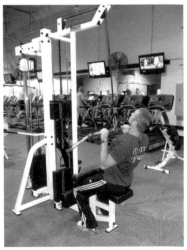

CLOSE GRIP LAT PULL-DOWN
At a lat pull down machine, after setting weight, grab bar with
close grip and sit down so butt and feet are firmly planted on the
seat and ground. Starting with arms extended pull bar towards
your chest as far as possible and slowly return to starting position.
Works: Latissimus Dorsi, mid back

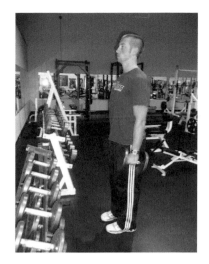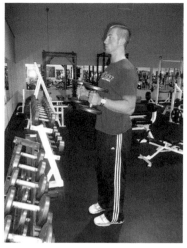

DUMBBELL HAMMER CURL
Start standing up tall with weights by side. Curls weights just like a normal curl but keep wrists in a neutral position. Do not swing weights.
Works: Biceps

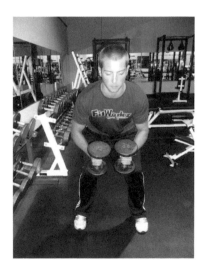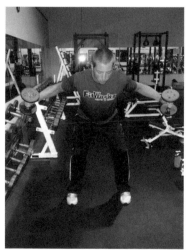

DUMBBELL BACK FLY
Stand with knees bent and torso flexed forward. Keep the head up and back straight. Weights should be above waist height with elbows bent. Lift the arms out to the sides up to shoulder height while squeezing the shoulder blades together. Keep elbows bent, engage core.
Works: Rhomboids, Middle Trapezius

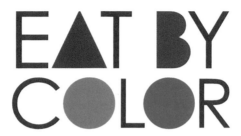

EAT BY COLOR

Do you want to learn even more about my
revolutionary weight loss plan? To obtain
FREE BONUS MATERIALS,
find us at:

facebook.com/EatbyColor

In health and wellness,

-Raymond M. Binkowski